STICKING TOGETHER

STICKING TOGETHER

Experiential Activities
for Family Counseling

written by

Jackie S. Gerstein, Ed.D.

College of Santa Fe
Western New Mexico University

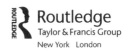

Routledge
Taylor & Francis Group
New York   London

First published by Accelerated Development

This edition published 2013 by Routledge

Routledge
Taylor & Francis Group
711 Third Avenue
New York, NY 10017

Routledge
Taylor & Francis Group
27 Church Road, Hove
East Sussex BN3 2FA

Routledge is an imprint of the Taylor & Francis Group, an informa business

STICKING TOGETHER: Experiential Activities for Family Counseling

A CIP catalog record for this book is available from the British Library.

Library of Congress Cataloging-in-Publication Data

Gerstein, Jackie S.
    Sticking together : experiential activities for family counseling
    / written by Jaclyn S. Gerstein.
       p. cm.
    Includes bibliographical references and index.
    ISBN 1-56032-864-9 (alk. paper)
    1. Family counseling. 2. Experiential psychotherapy. I. Title.
HQ10.G47 1999
362.82'86 – dc21   99-37021
                                      CIP

ISBN 1-56032-864-9 (paper)

CONTENTS

Foreword   ix
Introduction   xi

SECTION 1
The Foundations of Experiental Family Counseling   1

Experiential Counseling Defined / 1
Experiential Family Counseling Defined / 3
Characteristics of Experiential Family Counseling / 3
     Action-Centered / 4
     Strength-Promoting Program / 4
     Naturalistic Interactions / 4
     Use of Multifamily Groups / 5
     A Narrative Therapy Approach / 6
     The Focus on Play / 6
     The Developmental Needs of Children are Addressed / 7
The Functions of the Experiential Activities / 8
     Increasing Interest and Motivation for the Counseling Sessions / 8
     Reducing Resistance / 8
     Generating Additional Information / 9
     Acting as Metaphors for Family Problem Areas / 9
     Changing Family Patterns and Testing New Behaviors / 9
General Therapeutic Goals and Principles / 10
     Establishing Open and Honest Communication / 10
     Identifying Individual and Family Strengths / 11
     Developing a Solution-Focused Orientation / 11
     Modifying Family Roles / 12
     Having Fun as a Family / 12

SECTION 2
Setting Up An Experiential Program   13

Preparing for the Program / 13
     Selection of Family Participants and Program Orientation / 13
     The Family Performance Agreement / 14
     Family Performance Agreement / 15
     Participant Registration and Informed Consent Form / 17

Experiential Family Counseling Participant Registration
and Informed Consent Form / 19
Description of Problems and Goal Setting / 23
Goals of Experiential Family Counseling / 25
Inventory of Family Interests and Strengths / 25
The Experiential Counseling Program / 27
Using a Multisession Format / 27
Going to the Families / 27
Offering Services at Times Convenient for the Family / 27
Offering a Menu of Services / 28
Ongoing Assessment / 28
Follow-Up Strategies / 31
Follow-Up Contracts / 31
Progress Meetings / 31
Use of Adjunct Programs / 31

SECTION 3
Working with Different Age Groups

33

Special Issues of Young Children in Experiential Family Counseling / 34
Orientation / 34
Attention Span / 35
Physical and Verbal Skills / 35
Multi-family Groups / 36
Cultural Issues / 36
Challenged Children / 37
Summary / 37
Experiential Family Counseling with Adolescents / 38
Developmental Issues in Family Therapy with Adolescents / 38
Experiential Family Counseling with Adolescents / 38
Providing Opportunities for Leadership / 39
Positive Communication / 39
Power Struggles and Resistance / 40
Gender and Sexual Orientation / 40
Art & Music / 41
Humor / 41
Guiding Metaphor and Summary / 41

SECTION 4
The Counseling Session

43

Introduction/ Review Program Goals / 43
Physical and Emotional Safety Check / 43
PEEP: The Creation of Safe Space as a Norm in Experiential Family Counseling / 44
Introduction / 44
The PEEP Safety Check / 44
Framework / 45
P–Physical / 45
E–Emotional / 45
E–Environmental / 45
P–Personal / 45
Stop Mechanism / 46
Methodology / 46
Normalizing / 47

PEEP as an Intervention / 47
Summary / 47
The PEEP Safety Checklist / 49
Experiential Check-In Activities / 51
Movement Chain / 53
Musical Feelings / 55
Biblio Check-In / 57
Puppet Check-In / 59
Pick A Feeling / 61
Participant Rights and Responsibilities / 63
Participant Bill of Rights / 65
Participant Responsibilities / 66
Contracts / 67
The Family Contract / 69
The Behavioral Contract / 71
Acceptable/Unacceptable Behaviors Form / 73
Behavioral Family Contract / 75
A Sample Behavioral Family Contract / 77
Name Games and Warm-Ups / 79
Purpose / 79
Strategies / 79
Name Games / 81
Toss a Name / 81
Duck, Duck, Goose Name Game / 83
The Other Side Of the Blanket / 85
Family Have You Evers? / 87
Family Scavenger Hunt / 89
Penny for Your Thoughts / 91
Beach Ball Toss / 93
Family Jump Rope / 95
Family We-Play / 97
Make Beliefs: A Gift For & From Your Family / 99
Family-Building Initiatives / 101
Purpose / 101
Strategies for Selecting Family Building Initiatives / 101
Guidelines for Selecting Family-Building Initiatives / 103
Strategies for Using the Family-Building Initiatives / 104
Emphasize Physical and Psychological Safety / 104
Initially Use Initiatives to Break Down Barriers / 104
Focus on the Process / 104
Use Time-Outs / 104
End An Initiative When It Is Not Working / 104
Focus on Fun and Enjoyment / 104
Identify Family Strengths / 105
Use the Family-Building Initiatives as Metaphors / 105
Emphasize Solutions, Not Problems / 105
Identify and Disrupt Problematic Patterns / 106
Process the Family-Building Initiatives / 106
The Family Juggle / 107
The Nurturing Spoons / 109
Family Pick-Up Sticks / 113
Family Parts / 115
Family Knots / 117

The Family Jewels / 121
Family Tower of Power / 125
Chain Reaction / 127
The Family Strengths Protector / 129
The Family Obstacle Field / 133
Crossing the Problem Pit / 135
Crossing Over Hard Ships / 139
The Dumping Field / 143
T-Shirt Panorama / 147
Desert Island / 149
Review and Closure / 153
Purpose / 153
Strategies / 153
The Family Feelings Chart / 155
Structured Questionnaires / 157
Family Interaction Assessment / 159
Family Strengths Focus / 161
Expressive Arts Exercises for Review and Closure / 163
Nature Symbol / 163
The Family Crest / 163
The Family Fantasy World / 163
The Family Book / 163
Family Warm Fuzzies / 164
Bead Giving / 164
Word for the Day / 164
Follow-Up Contracts / 165
Contract With Ourselves . 167

Bibliography   **169**

Author Index   **171**

Subject Index   **173**

FOREWORD

There's a much interpreted Sufi folk tale about a blind man who is meeting an elephant for the first time. He touches the elephant's flowing, canvaslike ear and says, "Ah, an elephant is like a tree with huge broad leaves." Then he feels the elephant's short, curly tail and says, "No, the elephant is like a bristly, wild dog." Finally he holds the elephant's tubular trunk and exclaims, "Aha, I see, an elephant is like a giant muscular snake."

As mental health practitioners we are all, at first glance, blind to a family's central problem issues. The information we gather by just talking with family members can seem contradictory and confusing and, even more disconcerting, can take a great deal of time to sort through. Fortunately, Dr. Jackie Gerstein in *Sticking Together: Experiential Activities for Family Counseling*, provides us with an innovative and very effective treatment option.

Sticking Together contains solid theory on which experiential counseling is built, as well as specific activity planning guidelines, orientation games, family skill-building activities, and closure activities. Through these structured games, guided exercises, and processing activities, we can watch a family's sociodramas unfold before our eyes. The subtle interplays and obvious strategies family members use with one another come out into the open to be reinforced, challenged, or changed. By structuring the activities as metaphors for a family's identified problems, counselors can help family members practice solutions exquisitely tailored to their daily lives.

Dr. Gerstein has written a comprehensive, practical, enormously respectful handbook for mental health practitioners and the families in their care. Her vision serves us all.

Sherry Kaufield, MA, LCPC, ACHE

INTRODUCTION

Why experiential activities in a family counseling setting?

I studied family therapy during my doctoral program. Through my training, I got to conduct therapy in a traditional manner, in a regular office setting talking about the clients' problems as the primary mode of therapy. I'm not sure about the families' reactions, but I quickly got bored and tired of hearing families play verbal ping pong, blaming one another and other social systems for their problems. I became frustrated because the families were unhappy and stuck in unhealthy ways of doing things. And none of us seemed to know what to do about it. The families and I would watch the clock anticipating the end to our sessions.

I began to draw on my previous experience in wilderness and adventure therapy. I became more experiential during the counseling sessions, using games, art exercises, and adventure activities, combining my adventure-based counseling background with my family therapy training. I started working out these ideas with my staff at the psychiatric hospital where I was employed at the time. As we watched the families while they participated in the experiential activities, we engaged in an ongoing dialogue as to how to adapt the activities to make them more therapeutic and suitable for working with families.

Most families seemed to enjoy the sessions, and they reported positive changes, "I forgot how pleasurable it was spending time with my children." "My child has begun to listen to me for the first time in a long time," "My child is doing better in school." I also enjoyed the sessions and the families more.

Why a book on experiential activities for families?

I spoke with many family therapists who faced cognitive upheavals similar to those I had. They, too, were frustrated and unsatisfied with the more traditional counseling format. They came to understand, through their education and experience, that change most often occurs when the family is experiencing rather than just talking about the events in their life. The masters of family therapy—Erickson, Haley, Madanes, Whitaker, Satir—were naturally experiential during their therapy sessions. In fact, Whitaker's and Satir's techniques are generally categorized as experiential therapy.

Most family clinicians have the desire, but not enough tools and strategies to facilitate the family in experiencing. When given the tools to guide families through an experiential family counseling modality, most practitioners light up with excitement, as do the families whom they are counseling!

I believe that using experiential activities with families is good practice. I've been using these techniques with families for over 10 years. I still get excited watching families-in-counseling laugh, cry, and play together, watching them squeal with joy, furrow their brows as they work cooperatively to solve problems, and hug one another after the successful completion of an experiential exercise. I receive the great gift seeing families leave their counseling sessions feeling better about themselves as individuals and as family units.

Combining the experiential activities with the practices developed by family therapists is a powerful way to do therapy. I want to share these techniques with other practitioners. This book is one way for me to do so.

The Design of the Book

Sticking Together: Experiential Activities for Family Counseling is for the working practitioner. This book is meant to be used and reused, dogeared, written upon, misplaced, and dirtied. It comes in a convenient workbook format that easily allows readers to copy the forms, exercises and activities in order to use them again and again.

Section 1 provides some background information for using experiential activities with families. This section provides a basic understanding of the characteristics, functions, and goals of experiential family counseling. Clinicians, who are really serious about integrating an experiential approach into their everyday practices, are encouraged to do more reading on the topic and to develop their own theories and hypotheses as they observe this type of counseling in action.

Section 2 describes the skeleton of an experiential counseling program. Topics include selecting clients, using performance agreements and informed consent forms, facilitating goal setting, scheduling the counseling sessions, engaging in ongoing assessment, and designing follow-up strategies. Section 3 provides some strategies and techniques for working with specific populations, e.g., young children or adolescents.

The main section, Section 4, of the book presents the core of experiential counseling, the experiential exercises themselves. An extensive array of exercises and activities is provided. These include orientation materials, check-in activities, warm-up exercises, family-building initiatives (or exercises), and review exercises, as well as forms and contracts for families and practitioners to use.

The intent of this book is not to have practitioners take every idea presented at face value. *Sticking Together: Experiential Activities for Family Counseling* has been designed to plant some seeds of excitement towards experiential counseling. I hope that practitioners will question the concepts and activities, modify the material presented in the book to tailor it their own clinical settings, and develop their own strategies, techniques, and exercises depending on the families with whom they are working.

Special Thanks

I would like to thank several people connected directly or indirectly with this project. My colleagues from Oakwood Hospital, Sherry Kaufield, Joel Tucker, Sara Nash, and C.J. helped me dream up the creative ways to use the experiential activities with families. Three of the sections were written by the most brilliant clinicians I know—Sherry Kaufield, Stephanie Bryson and Juli Lynch. Sherry wrote the section entitled, "Special Issues of Young Children in Experiential Family Counseling." Stephanie describes some techniques for working with adolescents in "Experiential Family Counseling with Adolescents." Juli discusses the "Creation of Safe Space as a Norm in Experiential Family Counseling." Thanks also goes to Gina Griego, a favorite student of mine, who invented one of the new initiatives. Tim Julet, my editor from Accelerated Development, was of great assistance in helping me fine-tune the writing of this book. And finally, a special thanks goes to Mitchell, my brother, who taught me compassion and to all those family participants, who through their laughter and tears and through their struggles and affection, enriched my life.

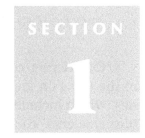

The Foundations of Experiental Family Counseling

The practices of family therapy and those of experiential counseling are being used in therapeutic settings throughout the world. However, combining these two approaches into the form of experiential family counseling presents a unique type of family intervention. This section assists the reader in gaining a theoretical foundation for using experiential counseling activities with families. Discussed are:

- □ Experiential Counseling Defined,
- □ Experiential Family Counseling Defined,
- □ Characteristics of Experiential Family Counseling,
- □ Functions of the Experiential Activities, and
- □ General Therapeutic Goals and Principles.

Experiential Counseling Defined

Experiential counseling, as described in this book, has its roots in adventure education, from the models developed by the Outward Bound Wilderness Programs and Project Adventure Challenge Ropes Courses (see writings by Kurt Hahn and Karl Rohnke for more information about these programs). With this counseling model, clients are facilitated through a series of physical and social tasks, where the need for problem-solving and communications provide situational analogies for problematic areas in their daily lives (Stitch, 1983). A classic example is the Human Knot whereby the counselor guides the group in creating a hand-in-hand human knot. The goal of the group is to get untangled without letting go of their hands. The need for problem-solving and communications becomes evident as the group members work toward their solution—a hand-in-hand circle with no tangles. The situational analogy can focus on any of a number of areas depending on the group's goals and needs—the characteristics of group entanglement or enmeshment, communication styles when people can see each other versus when they cannot, appropriate versus inappropriate physical touching, clearly giving directions, etc.

Experiential counseling is a holistic modality. Clients are asked to become involved in the tasks on mental, physical, emotional, and social levels. The experiential activities, which include trust-building activities, group goal-directed activities, and adventure challenge courses, are used to promote adaptive self-concept, internal locus of control, and problem-solving skills (Huber, 1997). The use of an activity-driven counseling modality promotes a more genuine and natural uncovering of a client's true personality, of the ways he tends to interact with others in his everyday life. These activities also tend to draw out clients' strengths and resources naturally.

Experiential counseling uses a cyclical model of learning whereby clients are asked to participate in an experiential exercise, reflect on the exercise, use new insights when engaging in the next experiential exercise, reflect on that, and so forth. This form of counseling is driven by the belief that change occurs when individuals engage in some activity, critically reflect upon the activity, derive some useful insight from the analysis, and incorporate the insight into some new understanding or behavior (Luckner & Nadler, 1997).

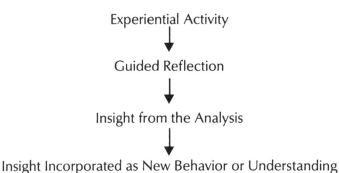

Experiential counseling differs from the more traditional talk therapies conducted in many clinical settings in that the client is a participant in counseling rather than a talker and listener (Wick, Wick, & Peterson, 1997). While many traditional talk therapies focus on introspective and analytical thinking through talking it out, experiential therapies focus on direct and concrete experiences followed by the analysis of these direct experiences. Instead of talking about experiences that are once or twice removed from the therapeutic setting, this sort of counseling examines the experiences that occur within the setting.

The experiential exercises often achieve levels of change that may be impossible to reach without such experiences (Gass & Scippa, 1990). Change almost always has some form of experience at its origin. Experiential counseling places the client close to that origin. This process is often more valuable for the transmission of knowledge than other forms of counseling (Gass, 1993). Underlying this philosophy is the notion that insight into one's areas of discomfort does not produce change in and by itself. Insight is valuable, and often offers a sense of ease and understanding for the client. But actual change requires a client to do something differently in her life. Change is an action-oriented process. Change can best occur from the process of translating insight into action through the active experiencing of new situations (Clapp & Rudolph, 1993, p. 113).

Experiential Family Counseling Defined

Experiential counseling that has traditionally been applied to individual and small group counseling is now being applied systematically to marriage and family counseling (Gillis & Gass, 1993). When experiential counseling is combined with family therapy, the treatment of the "identified client" becomes a family affair. The therapeutic interventions are designed not just for the client but for the identified client and her family. They all benefit directly from the experiential activities. The activities become metaphors for problem areas in a family's life, while family therapy techniques are used to ameliorate the family system.

Experiential family counseling is based on the philosophy and assumption that the family has the skills and resources for positive personal change and growth. The program activities, along with the accompanying family counseling, provide a powerful impetus for the utilization of the family's personal resources to achieve the desired changes. Family members gain new perspectives on their own abilities and their relationships with other family members.

Because of the experiential nature of the activities, the fronts, facades, and roles that families use to hide their nonworking behaviors become less effective. Instead of only talking about problem areas, the family sees its behaviors and interactional patterns demonstrated within the context of the activities. The counselors and family participants have the opportunity to observe the nonworking behaviors in action. The participants gain a better understanding of the consequences of their unhealthy and nonworking behavioral and interactional patterns. By designing activities which are metaphors for the family's problem areas, attitudes of learned helplessness, poor self-image, mistrust, and lack of self-confidence are replaced with self-confidence, self-efficacy, and a trusting of others, along with new and creative methods for solving the family's problems (Chase, 1981). The participants have the opportunity to practice new and alternative behaviors during the program activities. As a result of these positive changes, the family is better able to assist the identified client in getting his needs met within the family system.

Characteristics of Experiential Family Counseling

Several characteristics make experiential family counseling a powerful and unique therapeutic tool.

It is:

- action-centered, and
- strength-promoting.

It uses:

- naturalistic interactions,
- a multifamily group format,

☐ a narrative therapy approach,
☐ play to draw out a family's resources, and
☐ addresses the developmental needs of children and adolescents.

Action-Centered

As stated earlier, experiential family counseling is action-centered. Counseling becomes an active and multidimensional experience rather than a passive, talk-about analysis. The interactions among family members are observable and holistic. They involve affective, cognitive, and physical elements of each family member's personality. The counseling lends itself to examining the family's patterns and beliefs directly. "Clients are asked to 'walk' as well as 'talk' their behaviors during the therapeutic activity" (Gillis & Gass, 1993, p. 275).

The activities, the consequences related to the activities, and the reflection on the dynamics that occurred during the activity make learning more meaningful and real for the family members. The families get to establish new and, one hopes, healthier interactions within the counseling setting. This increases chances for transfer of learning to their settings outside of the therapeutic office.

Strength-Promoting Program

Experiential counseling stresses that both the counselor and the family focus on what is right in the family system. Efforts are made to try to sustain and protect that, rather than dwell on the family's' problem-saturated stories. The perspective adopted emphasizes that a strengths-based focus is much more useful for everyone (both clinician and clients) than one based on pathology and dysfunction (Buckley, Thorngren, & Kleist, 1997). The use of experiential activities in counseling demands that clinicians switch their perceptions from viewing clients as pathology-laden to viewing clients as needing a little assistance to tap into their resources (Gerstein, 1998).

> When we separate a person's or family's preferred experiences from the confines of a problem-saturated story, we find ourselves oriented toward inspiring histories, present strengths, and future dreams and hopes (Freeman, Epston, & Lobovits, 1997, p. 49).

The experiential activities are inherently designed to draw upon the family's strengths. Experiences and activities are presented to accent their strengths and abilities rather than their unhealthy coping behaviors. Families are challenged to shift from dwelling on limitations toward tapping into resources and strengths. The experiential activities ask individuals to view their lives from different angles and new perspectives in order to identify, examine, and draw upon those personal strengths and resources.

Naturalistic Interactions

During the experiential activities, the clinician and the family members themselves, obtain firsthand observations and assessments of family roles, communication patterns, problem-solving methods, and family interactions (Vass, Jacobs, & Slavek, 1984). A lot of information is gathered in a few hours of observing the family's interactions in these natural environments. This method avoids relying on secondhand talking about the problem.

This model also lends itself to integrating the interventions within the family's natural interactions as they occur. The family's interactional processes are stopped at periodic intervals, and the family members are asked to explore unhealthy consequences of their behaviors. The family begins to acknowledge and change destructive patterns by developing cues to interrupt these established response patterns. Opportunities are provided for families to attempt new alternatives to their more rigid, less effective interactional processes (Vass, Jacobs, & Slavek, 1984).

Use of Multifamily Groups

The experiential modality tends to be most effective when implemented as a multifamily group format—approximately two to four families per session. Multiple family group therapy is a deliberate, planned, psychosocial intervention with two or more families (Thorngren, Christensen, & Kleist, 1998). "Elements of education, combined with those of group process, have been implemented to harness the strengths of individual members and families to bring about greater problem-solving abilities for the group as a whole" (Thorngren et al., 1998, p. 125).

The benefits for using multifamily groups are numerous. First, the use of multifamily groups helps to reduce the defensiveness that is characteristic of families in trouble (Stanton, 1981). By identifying commonalities among the family groups, family members discover that their problems are not unique, and their defensiveness is reduced.

Second, the pressure typically placed on the clinician to produce change is diffused to a larger group of people (Stanton, 1981). A major responsibility of the participating families is to provide feedback and intervention strategies to the families. In other words, the families act as adjunct therapists for one another. Combining several families provides a way for enhancing "the natural helping elements so ingrained in most people" (Thorngren et al., 1998, p. 130).

Third, families often become socially isolated because of the self-perceived shame related to their family problems. Multifamily group counseling decreases the stigma associated with mental health services, thereby increasing opportunities for the engagement of at-risk families (Stone, McKay, & Stoops, 1996).

Finally, by participating in a multifamily group format, families can draw upon the strengths, objectivity, and role-modeling behaviors of a larger group of peers (Stanton, 1981). By observing other family groups during the experiential activities, families are given the opportunity to identify those positive roles, behaviors, and interactions that occur within the other families.

Testimonials from clinicians and clients have provided evidence of the efficacy of multifamily group counseling (Thorngren, et al., 1998). Rudolph (1997) conducted a qualitative study with four families who participated in a multifamily, experiential-based counseling program. The program participants reported that the multifamily group provided them with an opportunity to: (a) identify common areas of concern, (b) create bonding and support, and (c) "see themselves through a mirror image by watching other families in action" (p. 279).

A Narrative Therapy Approach

It is not within the scope of this book to provide an in-depth definition and explanation of the theory and approaches surrounding narrative therapy. Simply stated, though, narrative therapy is about helping people to tell their life stories in their own language. The clinician assists clients in telling their stories from a perspective that zeros in on their triumphs and courageousness rather than on their problems, difficulties and hopelessness. "These too-often bits of personal history can be the foundation for new, more healing life stories" (Simon, 1994, p. 6).

When the family members tell their stories, find new thoughts about old problems, imagine new endings for their future, they become creative, hopeful, and healthier. The chances for a good outcome to counseling improve. The block to success is verbal language. If counselors are to assist clients in reexamining and retelling their stories, then they need to learn the language of the client. "How can therapists, newly wed to the client family learn the foreign language and exotic legends of their clients rapidly enough to be effective?" (Riley, 1994, p. 21).

Experiential activities used within the counseling context can be used to create visible illustrations of the family story. Words become only part of the family's language and communication. Actions and behaviors become another part. Experiential family counseling can become the bridge between the invented reality of the family and the clinician's appreciation and understanding of the family's reality. Through the experiential activities, the family is provided the opportunity to act out their family story and, aided by their actions, to discover new, alternative endings to their legends. The experiential activities allow the family to look at their situation once removed from their normal day-to-day interactions. Discussing the experiential exercises stimulates the language and conversation of the family.

With more tools to work with than words alone, the clinician can assist the family in transforming their environment and in making the process more personal, more believable, and more securely anchored in their belief system. "There is a better chance to find new themes, new histories, create an alternative view of their problem, to invent a new reality. Fresh explanations that remove a negative label on the problem—to view the situation in a fresh light—lead to the process of change" (Riley, 1994, p. 35).

The Focus on Play

One of the major characteristics of the experiential counseling exercises is that they have an element of play and fun. From my experience working with families, I observed that most families reported that having fun and playing together was one of their most valuable lessons learned during the experiential activities. The benefits of using play in counseling are numerous and include some of the following.

First, play introduces fun and humor into a family system that may be experiencing severe stress and may have forgotten (or never known) how to enjoy one another (Eaker, 1994). Families seek counseling because the stress they are experiencing with one another is too high for them to cope with on their own. With play, families laugh together, touch one another, connect on levels that only humor and fun can facilitate. Stress is reduced. Mental, emotional, physical, and spiritual health is enhanced. The act of the family playing together and enjoying one another's company may be the healthiest therapeutic component of their counseling experience.

Second, play assists family members in creating a space where creative problem-solving can occur. Developing playful experiences in troubled families is often a first step in creating a safe and secure environment necessary to change and grow (Quereau, 1993). Family members can retreat into the play if anxiety escalates and/or when issues surface at a time when the family is not ready to deal with them (Eaker, 1994).

The Developmental Needs of Children are Addressed

If one were to walk into family counseling sessions around the world, the following scene would be viewed over and over again. The family comes into the room and sits on the sofa. The clinician asks the family how their week has been. Mom or dad answers. The children begin to fidget. The clinician gives the children paper and crayons and requests that they color in the corner of the room.

Clinicians cannot be totally faulted for this. Many family counselors have not been trained to create interventions that take into account the developmental needs of children. In recent times, much of the family therapy literature and training has focused on abstract theories and has neglected the nitty-gritty concerns of clinical work. Even family counselors, who are motivated to include children, often do not feel confident about how to do so, given the lack of literature and techniques, and the variety of ages, presenting problems, and family configurations seen in practice (Green in Gil, 1994, Introduction).

If true family counseling is the ultimate goal, children need to be considered as equal partners in the therapeutic process, and this process needs to be adapted accordingly. When family counseling includes children, the clinician needs to use techniques that not only take into account the developmental characteristics of the children, but also techniques that use the unique strengths, insights, and healthy behaviors that the children bring into the counseling setting. Serious discussion and methodical problem-solving often impose on children's communication, shutting out their voices, and inhibiting their special abilities, knowledge, and creative resources (Freeman, Epston, & Lobovits, 1997). The experiential exercises provide an environment where children can communicate in languages that are more natural to them—through play, art, and body gestures. A more natural and real representation of the child's perspective about the family is reflected. The children's world and their language is welcomed and encouraged in a way that indicates they are elicited as helpers in the counseling process. "Through having a different kind of conversation about a problem or playing with us in fantasy, the child often finds a 'solution' we could never have anticipated" (Freeman, Epston, & Lobovits, 1997, p. 7).

The use of experiential exercises becomes a gentler approach for children than the talking therapies. In this context, children view counseling as a time to have fun, not a time to get help. Furthermore, experiential counseling "does not require highly developed verbal or cognitive abilities, because the children experience the interventions 'in their bones', not in their heads" (Wick, Wick, and Peterson, 1997, p. 56). Section 3 of this book addresses special issues and techniques when working with children in an experiential family counseling setting.

The Functions of the Experiential Activities

The previous information described the more general characteristics of an experiential family counseling program. This topic area zeros in on the specific functions of the experiential exercises themselves, as they serve several functions that are unique to action-oriented therapies. The functions include:

- ☐ Increasing interest and motivation for the counseling sessions,
- ☐ Reducing resistance,
- ☐ Generating additional information,
- ☐ Acting as metaphors for family problem areas, and
- ☐ Changing family patterns and testing new behaviors.

Increasing Interest and Motivation for the Counseling Sessions

Experiential exercises often lead to increased interest and motivation for the counseling sessions. By their very nature, these exercises are both enticing and engaging. They "offer an escape from the humdrum experience of doing the same thing session after session, a practice that, at best, shuns creativity" (Rosenthal, 1998, p. 4). A typical client statement about experiential counseling is, "I do not know what to expect each time I come to counseling, and this makes it exciting for me."

Clients' unfamiliarity with experiential activities also causes them to be placed outside their comfort areas and into states of dissonance and disequilibrium. Because of these states, clients are motivated to develop different and often more adaptive coping and problem-solving skills. They are provided with new and unique experiences to explore new understandings of themselves (Wick et al., 1997).

Reducing Resistance

The experiential exercises are helpful in bypassing the family's resistance. An atmosphere of playfulness often reduces resistances and defenses. The playful nature of the exercises help decrease the anxiety typically associated with therapeutic settings (Miller, 1994). Eliciting family concerns and problems in the context of play and games allows them to be examined once removed from the real problem. Both problems and strengths are seen from new perspectives as resistances are dropped.

Generating Additional Information

The experiential exercises provide additional assessment information about the family. Diagnostic information is gathered without relying strictly on verbal interviews (Irwin & Malloy, 1994). The family members act out their family stories with words and actions rather than with just words.

Through participation in the exercises, both the family members and the clinician can directly observe family interactions such as who speaks to whom, who is in alliance with whom, who makes the decisions, who is excluded, who is included, and so forth. This information either confirms or challenges the family's perceptions about their interactions and relationships.

Acting as Metaphors for Family Problem Areas

The experiential exercises act as metaphors for the family's problem areas. The activities allow family members, especially children, to express themselves metaphorically with play within the context of the exercise, a less intimidating prospect than verbal enactment (Miller, 1997). Because games and play are seen as less threatening than serious verbal discourse, family members often use the exercises as a way to uncover and express their family-based concerns.

The exercises inherently elicit the family's typical behavioral patterns and interactions—interactions that may be masked in other therapeutic settings. The clinician strategically selects exercises that have themes resembling a problem that the family wants to examine and change. Asking family members to view their problem areas in the form of a game-like metaphor makes it easier for the family to deal with than trying to solve the problem head-on.

Changing Family Patterns and Testing New Behaviors

The experiential exercises are designed to change both the presenting family patterns and the underlying interactional sequences that surround them. As the families participate in a number of exercises, repetitive patterns of interaction are discovered. Once identified, the repetition of unhealthy sequences and interactions is prevented through the introduction of alternatives during the program activities.

Family members are provided with a safe and permissive environment to experiment with new behaviors. Action-oriented interventions are introduced into the experiential activities as family members interact with one another. These interventions are designed to interrupt and break rigid patterns of doing, thinking, and feeling while family members are engaged in the activity.

A case example of the Low family exemplifies the functions just discussed. The family came to counseling due to reported difficulties with their older son. The family consisted of mother, father, older son, and younger son. They were asked to participate in Crossing the Problem Pit (see page 135 for a description). On the problem pit runway, they listed problems such as son's smoking, money problems, sons fighting, and so forth, until at the end of the pit, they jotted down the phrase "Dad's drinking." They were asked to cross the pit using the boards (again see description). According to the directions, if any family member fell off the board and touched into the pit, they were to start again. The family progressed smoothly until they got towards the end of the pit and were ready to cross over Dad's drinking. A family member fell off the board and touched into the pit. The family was asked to begin again. The second time the same scenario occurred. The family reached Dad's drinking and a member touched into the pit. This same scene was repeated four times! At that point, the family was asked to gather in a sitting circle on the floor and talk about what was happening. Dad's drinking was the topic, and this was the first time it was discussed by the family.

First of all, the family was engaged fully in the activity. Because the family consisted of older and younger adolescent males, the potential to lose them through talking therapy was high. Second, resistance was obviously reduced as the family, for the first time, identified Dad's drinking as a problem. Third, additional information was generated through the writing out of problems on the problem-pit runway and through watching the family interact as they attempted (unsuccessfully) to cross the problem pit. Fourth, the problem pit obviously became a metaphor for the difficulties the family members were having with Dad's drinking behavior. Finally, patterns were changed and the family members got to test new behaviors when they sat down to discuss Dad's drinking for the first time.

Because these functions are quite specific to the experiential counseling activities, the clinician needs to insure that she takes advantage of these functions and uses them to their fullest potential. A huge therapeutic moment would have been lost if the clinician had not asked the family to examine the difficulties they had crossing over the problem of Dad's drinking.

General Therapeutic Goals and Principles

This final topic of the foundation section specifies some general therapeutic goals and principles for families participating in this form of counseling. Even though each participating family develops specific goals for their own experiential counseling sessions (see Section 4, Description of Problems and Goal Setting, for more information), experiential counseling focuses on some general goals for all families who become involved in the program. These are:

- ☐ Establishing honest and open communication,
- ☐ Identifying individual and family strengths,
- ☐ Developing a solution-focused orientation,
- ☐ Modifying family role assignments, and
- ☐ Having fun as a family.

Establishing Open and Honest Communication

On top of the list is the opening of communication lines between the family members. The achievement of the family's goals is dependent upon the family members' ability to communicate needs, desires, concerns, and affection. "Participation in an emotionally-charged, adventure-based experience where vulnerabilities are shared and risks are taken may enhance communication and promote family intimacy" (Rudolph, 1997, p. 279).

> "Me and my mom cooperated. I listened to her."
> A 15-year-old daughter from a family
> consisting of just her and her mom.
> They argued intensely and often.

Identifying Individual and Family Strengths

During the experiential counseling sessions, the counselor and the family members accentuate the strengths of each family member and the family unit. Areas of family competence are identified and highlighted (Stanton & Todd, 1982). A question often asked after the completion of an experiential exercise is "What allowed your family to be successful during the exercise?" During the processing and debriefing of the exercises, the family members are guided in using these strengths to solve family-related problems. Through identifying and building upon individual and family strengths, current functional behaviors are supported and built upon (Eastwood, Sweeney, & Piercy, 1987).

> "It taught us to interdepend on one another and that there are a lot of things we
> can't do individually, but as a family we can."
> A father in a family of four with two adolescent
> girls, one of whom had several residential
> placements due to substance abuse.

Developing a Solution-Focused Orientation

The family is encouraged to shift from a problem-centered, problem-focused perspective to one that emphasizes a present and future orientation (Eastwood et al., 1987). Participating families are given an opportunity to interact in novel ways, creating new behaviors and unique outcomes that often contradict their unhealthy interactional patterns (Rudolph, 1997).

During the experiential exercises, families are asked to generate a large spectrum of outcomes and solutions to problem situations. The family is taught, experientially, that when problems do develop in the future, they will have available a wide range of solution-based options (Eastwood et al., 1987). When the families believe that they have the solutions and resources available to solve problems, future problems may not seem so overwhelming. They develop a positive expectation that they will be able to generate current and future solutions (Eastwood et al., 1987).

> "We got to look at different ways of doing things rather than doing it the same
> old way."
> A single mother of one adolescent
> girl and two preadolescent boys.

Modifying Family Roles

Families in distress often need to develop more flexible behavioral repertoires so that they can respond more effectively to developmental needs of individual family members, especially those of the children (Stanton & Todd, 1982). Parents need to learn to tolerate new and often unpredictable family situations that typically arise when their child reaches a new developmental stage (Davis, 1987).

Both the multigroup format and the experiential activities encourage the development of more flexible family roles. Parents often need to develop adaptive behavioral responses when working through the novel experiential exercises with their children. One of more significant discoveries from Rudolph's (1997) research was the realization by the parents that their children had good ideas. The experiential activities "called on family members to work cooperatively, leaving behind family roles and allowing for opportunities for role flexibility" (Rudolph, 1997, p. 279).

Throughout the counseling, the parents are assisted in correcting, if indicated, the family hierarchical system. When the child is living in the home, it is developmentally appropriate for the parents to be in charge (Stanton & Todd, 1982). Several of the experiential exercises (see The Family Obstacle Field as an example) have been designed to enhance the boundary around the youth by giving the parents tasks to create hierarchical boundaries between them and the child (Fishman, Stanton & Roseman, 1982). Both parental and child roles then become more solid and defined.

> "It was nice to have my dad give me directions."
> A 16-year-old girl who had four residential
> placements prior to the program.

Having Fun as a Family

Families with problems often have forgotten how to have fun with one another. The playful and fun nature of many of the experiential activities facilitate family members' enjoyment in being with one another. In fact, the fun that typically occurs during program activities tends to be the highlight for most of the participating families.

> "It has been a long time since we have played together. We saw that we can still play together."
>
> A blue collar working father, who works
> two jobs to support his wife and three
> kids. He said this with tears in his eyes.

Setting Up
An Experiential Program

This chapter contains suggestions about those preparatory, programming, and follow-up strategies that can be used to achieve the mission and goals of a family counseling program that uses experiential activities. It provides the general and larger framework for the actual experiential counseling sessions.

Preparing for the Program

Selection of Family Participants and Program Orientation

The counselor should develop a set of criteria to use when considering a family for this type of counseling. McHardy and Root (1992), who operated an agency that provided family experiential programs for seven years, found this type of counseling modality most suitable for families who:

☐ have had specific family life cycle difficulties (e.g., blended families, adoptive families, foster families, grieving families, families experiencing developmental crises),

☐ are verbally intimidated in a traditional counseling environment,

☐ are traditionally resistant,

☐ desire an alternative enrichment experience,

☐ need support and networking opportunities to overcome isolation, and/or

☐ desire an assessment tool to observe and comment upon the nature of their interaction over a period of time.

Because experiential-based counseling programs are unique in their format and philosophy, each program using this modality should establish some participant selection criteria. The following general guidelines are recommended for family eligibility in a program that offers experiential family counseling activities:

- ☐ children a minimum of seven years old (I have successfully run this program with 3- and 4-year-olds, but it takes a little extra effort and activity adaptation),
- ☐ no active suicidal or violent behaviors,
- ☐ a commitment of all family participants to attend all sessions,
- ☐ an openness to learn about and improve family interactions, and
- ☐ parent(s) should have some minimal skills for managing their children (Clapp & Rudolph, 1993).

To address the issue of informed consent, every potential family candidate receives an orientation to clarify the purpose of the experiential activities and to determine if the program is appropriate for that potential family participant. The orientation addresses the program format, the goals of the program, possible risks, why the program can be important to the family, and how the skills learned in the program can be pertinent to issues in their home environment. It is important that the family has a clear understanding of the nature of the program before making a commitment.

The counselor and the family discuss whether there is a match between what the family wants and what the program can provide (Clapp & Rudolph, 1993). The orientation is designed to determine if the family's areas of concern can be met by this type of program, if there is a fit between the family's problem areas/concerns and the goals of the experiential programming.

Following the orientation, the counselor and the family members decide whether or not the program is appropriate for that family. The family needs to be motivated about their participation and should choose to participate voluntarily. The counselor needs to believe that this type of intervention can have therapeutic benefits for that family.

The Family Performance Agreement

Once a mutual decision to participate in the program has been made by the counselor and family, a Family Performance Agreement can be developed. The Family Performance Agreement explicitly states in writing the expectations, program services, participant responsibilities, and time commitments. It acts as a written informed consent and helps avoid misconceptions and misunderstandings about the nature of the program. A sample agreement can be found on the following page.

Family Performance Agreement

Program Activities

We have been informed about the nature of the program. We fully realize that this is a therapeutic program and not a recreational one. We understand that we may be asked to participate in any or all of the following activities:

- ☐ Experiential exercises,
- ☐ Expressive arts exercises,
- ☐ Team building initiatives,
- ☐ Adventure ropes courses,
- ☐ Debriefing/Processing sessions, and
- ☐ Multifamily group counseling sessions.

Program Services

The program staff will provide the following services to participating families:

- ☐ A Program orientation,
- ☐ Program activity skill instruction,
- ☐ Supervision and emergency medical care,
- ☐ Group and family counseling, and
- ☐ Family evaluations.

Participant Responsibilities

We agree to adhere to the following rules while participating in the program activities:

- ☐ We will abide by any special rules and regulations developed to ensure the health, safety, and welfare of the participants;
- ☐ We will not carry any knives, blades, or firearms;
- ☐ We will refrain from the use of illegal substances and/or alcohol during the counseling activities;
- ☐ We will refrain from becoming involved in any physical confrontations that can cause bodily harm to self or others;
- ☐ We agree to replace or pay for any property damage or loss due to negligence or acting-out behavior;
- ☐ Cigarette smoking by minors is allowed only with parental permission (Smoking periods will be set by staff); and
- ☐ Respectful language is to be used by all participants.

Family Commitment

With the above knowledge in mind, we voluntarily agree to:

      ☐   Attend all sessions and complete the program time commitment,
      ☐   Try everything to the best of our ability, and
      ☐   Cooperate with our family, the staff, and other families.

Upon acceptance and admission into the program, we the _____ family, agree to commit to the program and follow the procedures outlined in this contract for a time period beginning on __/__/__ and terminating __/__/__.

Signatures of Family Members:

_____   _____

_____   _____

Signatures of Program Staff:

_____   _____

Participant Registration and Informed Consent Form

The ethical guidelines of the American Counseling Association state that the counselor must inform the client of the purposes, goals, techniques, and limitations of the counseling services. The American Psychological Association's Code of Ethics states that clients are to be fully informed as to the purpose and nature of treatment procedures and must freely acknowledge that participants have freedom of choice as to participation.

The Participant Registration and Informed Consent Form is the document that acts as an informed consent. It serves two major purposes. First, it insures that the family understands their risks and rights in the program, and second, it provides some measure of legal protection for the counselor.

The major sections of the Participant Registration and Informed Consent Form are:

- ☐ participant information,
- ☐ background information,
- ☐ the use of audio-visual recording,
- ☐ understanding of risk,
- ☐ waiver of legal claims,
- ☐ authorization for medical treatment for a minor, and
- ☐ acknowledgement of voluntary participation.

Parents or guardians of children under 18 years of age need to sign the form. The parent and child are asked fill out the child's form together while the parent explains the key points to the child. A sample form follows.

Experiential Family Counseling Participant Registration and Informed Consent Form

Participant's Name: _____ Date:_____

Address: _____ City: _____State: ___ Zip:_____

Telephone #: _____ Date of Birth:_____

Sex: ____Male ____Female   Height: _____ Weight: _____

Name of Person To Be Notified in Case of Emergency:_____

Address of Emergency Contact: _____

City: _____ State: _____ Zip: _____

Telephone #: _____ Relationship: _____

Background Information

Experiential Family Counseling is an action-oriented approach to counseling. Family clients may be asked to become engaged in a series of mentally and physically challenging activities such as cooperative games, trust building activities, problem-solving initiative activities, and expressive arts activities. During and following the activities, discussions or debriefings focus on seeing and understanding communication patterns, family relationships, problem-solving techniques, and areas of competence.

Use of Audio-Visual Recordings

In order to provide quality services, photographs or video recordings, or both, may be taken of the family sessions. These photographs and tapes are used as part of the program. The families and the staff may review these photographs or tapes as a means for exploring family interactions and behaviors. Photographs and videotapes of the family may be given to the family as part of the program format. Other photographs or videotapes will be destroyed following the family's involvement in the program upon the family's request. The photographs or videotapes will not be used for any other purposes without the family's written permission on a separate release form.

Understanding of Risk

You may be asked to take emotional, physical, and mental risks. You do not need physical prowess to participate in the experiential activities. The physical and emotional safety of participants is always of the utmost and primary concern of the facilitators. Individuals are always given a choice as to their degree of participation.

The type of possible risks that may occur during the sessions vary significantly from participant to participant. The following lists identify those risks that have been described by past participants.

Physical

- [ ] running, jumping, stretching, lifting,
- [ ] inability to physically complete tasks,
- [ ] trusting one's physical safety to others, and
- [ ] physically touching others.

Emotional

- [ ] disclosing personal feelings,
- [ ] asking for help and assistance,
- [ ] expressing feelings of afftection anger, fear,
- [ ] looking silly in front of others,
- [ ] providing and receiving emotional support, and
- [ ] giving and receiving positive and negative feedback.

I recognize and acknowledge that by participating in the experiential-based counseling sessions, there are certain physical and emotional risks. I understand that the utmost care and attention will be given to the health and safety of the participants. I agree to assume and accept the full risk of any injuries, illnesses, damages, or loss which I may sustain as a result of my participation in any and all activities connected with or associated with the experiential-based counseling sessions.

I understand that I should be free of any physical, medical, and/or mental conditions that may create undue risk to myself or others who may depend on me. If in doubt, I will seek medical advice before my participation in the experiential-based counseling sessions. I also agree to inform the facilitators of any situation(s) that may be a danger to myself or my coparticipants. These situations may include feeling sick or very tired, and having difficulty performing a skill.

As a participant in the Experiential Family Counseling sessions, I also agree to abide by any established rules and regulations set forth by the staff and understand that failure to comply with these rules may result in my removal from the session.

Parent Permission and Authorization for Medical Care

(To be completed by the parent/guardian, if participant is under 18 years of age)

I give my child, _____, permission to participate in the experiential-based counseling sessions. I fully understand the nature of the activities and objectives of the program. I am aware of the physical and mental demands as described in the Background Information and Understanding and Assumption of Risk sections. I grant consent for my child to participate in the program activities.

To the best of my knowledge, my child, _____, is physically and mentally able to participate in the experiential-based counseling sessions. Should my child become ill or injured, I give permission for the program staff to render first aid and to seek emergency medical and rescue services for my child. I acknowledge that any medical and accident insurance I consider necessary will be my responsibility to locate and purchase.

To the Participant:

I have read and understand the Background Information and the Understanding of Risk. I understand the nature of the program activities. I am voluntarily choosing to participate in the program activities. I have carefully read this agreement and understand its contents, and I sign it of my own free will.

Signature of Participant: _____

Date:_____

To the Parent (if participant is under 18 years of age):
I have read and understand the Background Information, Understanding of Risk, Parent Permission, and Authorization for Medical Care. I understand the nature of the program activities. I have carefully read this agreement and understand its contents, and I sign it of my own free will.

Signature of Parent: _____

Date: _____

Description of Problems and Goal Setting

After the family makes a commitment to participate in the program, the counselor interviews the family members to explore their most significant concerns. The counselor asks each family member to express her opinion on the issues and concerns that she would like to see addressed during the experiential family counseling sessions (Davis, 1987; Haley, 1976). The family members' description should include clear, concrete data about the life difficulties that brought the family into counseling. Involvement by each member of the social unit is sought. This process gives all family members the message that everyone will be given the opportunity and will be expected to participate in the counseling sessions (Haley, 1976).

From this information, goals are set for the counseling sessions. Bill O'Hanlon (1994) and Insoo Kim Berg (1994) have suggestions for goal setting with families.

Goal Setting Recommendations from the Writings of Bill O'Hanlon (1994)

- ☐ Work towards resolving the concern that brought the family into counseling.
- ☐ Include how often, when (date/time/deadline), and how long the goal will be implemented.
- ☐ Ensure that all the family members agree that the goal is relevant and achievable.
- ☐ Set an expectancy of a successful outcome.
- ☐ "Negotiate achievable goals in videotalk, in terms of actions or results that could be seen and heard on a videotape" (p. 48).
- ☐ Create subgoals that will indicate progress towards the major goal.

Goal Setting Recommendations from the Writings of Insoo Kim Berg (1994)

- ☐ Goals must be important to all participating family members.
- ☐ Goals must be small enough and simple enough to be achievable.
- ☐ Goals emphasize healthy family interactions.
- ☐ Goals are stated as gaining something rather than omitting something, as beginning healthy behaviors rather than ending unhealthy ones.

One way to facilitate goal-setting is to tell families what other families have expressed as beneficial outcomes due to their involvement in an experiential program. A worksheet such as the one on the following page can give families suggestions about those potential outcomes and goals for their counseling program.

Goals of Experiential Family Counseling

Directions: Check off one or two goals that you believe are important for your family to work on during the experiential counseling sessions.

__ To become a more caring, responsible family unit.

__ To develop techniques for the healthy release of emotions.

__ To increase the family's skills in problem-solving and conflict resolution.

__ To develop more open and honest communication lines between the family members.

__ To identify and build upon the family's strengths that support current functional and healthy behaviors.

__ To increase the family's ability to have fun with one another and enjoy one another's company.

__ To shift from a problem-centered, problem-focused perspective to one which emphasizes present and future successes.

__ To assist the family in correcting the family hierarchical system (e.g., having the parent(s) in charge of the family).

__ To help family members respond more effectively to developmental needs of each family member.

Inventory of Family Interests and Strengths

Along with obtaining information about the presenting concerns, the counselor gathers information about the family's perceptions of their strengths and interests. Each family member is asked to describe those family qualities that he believes is beneficial to the family, those qualities he would like the family to possess, and those family characteristics that are satisfactory and pleasurable (Eastwood, Sweeney, & Piercy, 1987). The counselor should explore the family apart from their problems. The focus should be on each family member's interests, unique qualities, and ideas for positive change (Freeman, Epston, and Lobotvits, 1997).

> Such discoveries can become the foundation upon which an alternative story is built, one based upon the child's and family's competencies and sufficiently compelling to stand up against the problem-dominated story (Freeman, Epston, & Lobotvits, 1997, p. 35).

Questions that may elicit this type of information include:

- ☐ Can I take some time to get to know you all without the problem, so that I can first respect you as individuals and as a family?
- ☐ Can you tell me about some of the abilities, interests, and special qualities of (the family member) that you especially appreciate?
- ☐ What makes you unique and special?
- ☐ What would you like me to know about you or (the family member) aside from how the problem is affecting you/her/him?
- ☐ What are your hopes and dreams?
- ☐ What can you tell me about your family relationships apart from the problem (Freeman, Epston, & Lobovits, 1997)?

Information gathered from this type of questioning is used to help design the counseling sessions. The counseling sessions are tailored to the family. Activities are selected and introduced that draw upon and accent their interests, strengths, and hopes.

The Experiential Counseling Program

This section describes the general logistics of the experiential counseling program. The following sections provide a more detailed description of the structure of the counseling sessions and types of activities and exercises that can be used during the sessions.

There are several practices that can be used to make the experiential family counseling format more accessible and inviting. These include:

- ☐ using a multisession format
- ☐ going to families
- ☐ offering services at times convenient for the families
- ☐ offering a menu of services.

Using a Multisession Format

Many experiential programs offer one-day, intensive experiences. Single event approaches to this type of counseling with distressed families can do more harm than good (Gillis & Gass, 1991).

It is recommended that the use of experiential family counseling be structured over multiple sessions over several weeks or months. Rudolph (1997) recommends, "Use a multi-session, program format [. . .] to allow sufficient time for families to work through the phase of enactment of family difficulties to the phase of intervention as family members become empowered to actively do something different" (p. 282).

Going to the Families

Many experiential programs operate sites and facilities that are quite a distance from the communities where the families live, and families are asked to come to these facilities. This may be a problem not only because of the distance that needs to be traveled, but also because it is more threatening for the family to go to a strange and unfamiliar environment.

One solution is to offer community-based programs. Experiential programs can be introduced in local school gymnasiums, church basements, or community centers. An even more "go-to-the families" approach can be introduced where the counselor brings the experiential activities to the families in their own homes.

Offering Services at Times Convenient for the Family

The meeting location, the meeting times, and length of sessions are worked out collaboratively with the family. Programs have to be offered at times convenient for the families. Meeting times would be based on the family's availability. Evenings or weekends will probably best meet the family's time constraints. Practitioners must be willing to meet with families during their (the families') free hours. Attempts are made to establish a once-a-week or twice-a-month schedule.

The optimal session length is two to three hours. This time frame:

☐ meets most families schedules,
☐ meets the developmental needs of younger children and older adults, and
☐ allows enough time to introduce and process an experiential activity.

Families attend from three to eight sessions depending on family motivation, therapeutic goals, and logistical factors (e.g., predetermined length of program, financial concerns, transportation).

Offering a Menu of Services

The counseling activities should be designed around the desires and interests of the participating families. Because of the large array of experiential activities, families can be given the opportunity to help design their program. The practitioner can work collaboratively with the participating family to decide the types of experiential activities (e.g., high physical vs. low physical demands, more talking vs. less talking, fun vs. serious activities), the time frames (i.e., evenings, weekends, length of sessions, number of sessions), and types of desired processing and debriefing activities (e.g., discussions, art activities, writing exercises, dramatics).

Given the working principle that the practitioner/family relationship is collaborative, families should have a say in the types of experiential activities in which they would like to participate. They can be given a menu of sorts: physical or not physical activities? cognitively challenging? fun and goofy? strong use of verbal skills? use of art activities? Because a family may be unsure about the types of activities that they enjoy or desire, the facilitator can introduce different sorts of activities, and make note of those that best match the family's interests, desires, motivations, and needs (Gerstein, 1997).

The practitioner's role is to elicit and take as much of what the family members present to design the activities around the family members. Family members are the experts about themselves. The facilitator is the expert in program design. It becomes the peg-in-the-hole philosophy. The goal isn't to form the family into a round peg so they can fit in the round hole (unless they explicitly state that this is their goal). The designers make the hole fit their shape. If the underlying mission is to address the family's unique personality and to empower them to have some direction in their life, then all opportunities should be provided for them to do so (Gerstein, 1997).

Ongoing Assessment

Because experiential counseling is an ongoing and evolving process, assessment is also ongoing and evolving. Many of the experiential exercises are designed to gain further information about the problems affecting the family. Many problems a family may be experiencing are beyond their immediate awareness. The nature of the experiential exercises brings them to the forefront. The experiential exercises are valuable assessment tools because families are asked to interact with one another in unfamiliar activities. Because of this unfamiliarity, families often project their behavior patterns, personalities, family interaction patterns, and interpretations into the activities (Gillis & Gass, 1993).

A family's story tends to change form as it emerges during the experiential exercises. The facilitator must always remain cognizant of what the family is saying and mold the experiential exercises and processing sessions around the family's emerging story.

An ongoing informal assessment can include the following questions.

☐ Do the experiential exercises and related processing sessions directly relate to the family's unique personality and their current concerns?
☐ Is each family member getting an opportunity to tell his or her story?
☐ Is the family identifying both healthy and unhealthy interactional sequences?
☐ Are opportunities being provided for the family to draw upon and utilize their strengths and resources?

Based on the answers to these questions, the experiential exercises and related processing sessions are continually selected, created, modified, adapted, and rejected with the counselor's flexibility being the key to the effective use of this assessment information (Gerstein, 1997).

Follow-Up Strategies

Follow-up sessions and strategies should be used to consolidate and reinforce the changes and gains families have made during the counseling sessions. Once the family has begun to make these positive changes, methods need to be implemented that reinforce these changes to prevent the reoccurrence of negative behaviors and to enhance clients' ability to adapt to new conflicts. Experiential counseling programs without follow-up experiences lack the strength of interventions with follow-up strategies (Gillis & Gass, 1993). Follow-up techniques such as contracts, progress meetings, and adjunct services can support the family as they transfer learning from the counseling environment to their home environment.

Follow-Up Contracts

The follow-up contract specifies a plan to deal with future problems, problems similar to the ones that brought the family into therapy (Eastwood, Sweeney, & Piercy, 1987). The contract describes those steps that the family will take to solve future problems. The first steps are based on techniques to prevent future incidents. In additional steps, the family specifies those actions they will take if a problem occurs. A sample Follow-Up Contract can be found in the Review and Closure section of this book.

Progress Meetings

Progress meetings can be planned for the family to meet with the counselors and the other participating families at regular, prespecified intervals following program termination. The progress meeting serves as a check-in. It becomes a type of support group, whereby the family can discuss and elicit feedback regarding progress, set-backs, and strategies for living as a healthy family. Continued check-up visits can occur every 4–6 weeks to monitor the progress of the change process.

Use of Adjunct Programs

Adjunct programs may be recommended to the family groups based on their needs and problems. Problems within the family may require some additional treatment that experiential family counseling cannot provide. Family problems may be severe enough to indicate some longer term family therapy. If this is the case, the family is referred to an agency which would be able to provide this type of treatment. Self-help support groups such as Alcoholics Anonymous, Ala-Teen, Alanon, or Parents Without Partners can also be recommended to assist the family with some needed external supports.

Working with Different Age Groups

When properly implemented, experiential-based counseling can address the developmental needs of both young children and adolescents. Based on the age of the children in the participating family and their goals, adjustments need to be made in the way the experiential activities are selected, introduced, and facilitated. This section provides some tips for working with different age groups.

Special Issues of Young Children in Experiential Family Counseling

Sherry Kaufield, MA, LCPC, ACHE

Working with young children in experiential family programs can be very challenging, but the results can be wonderfully interesting and extremely productive. Often the most flexible person in a family system controls the system (Madanas, 1981). Young children are experts at being flexible. If they do not get what they want in one way, they will simply find another way to reach their goals. Their family role can become that of catalyst, antagonist, attention diverter, unifier, demotivator or any combination of these or many other roles. They often function (consciously or not) much like an atom's nucleus, around which other crucial components (family members), establish loops and patterns.

When a child's role becomes clarified during the experiential activities, the family has a chance to really focus on the family system issues that brought them into counseling. These include the dynamics created by the child's wants and needs. This is not to say that the child in a family system is more significant that any other family member, or that determining a child's role should be the focus of counseling. Each and every person is a critical part of the dynamic that defines a family. Children just have a unique way of seeing family issues, deflecting or solidifying them, by the very nature of their dependency and family position (Satir, 1964). When they are involved in the counseling process, getting to the core of these issues is clearly enhanced.

One of the counselor's goals is to get as complete a picture as possible of how all individual family members give and take, initiate and respond, define themselves and are defined by one another. The main challenge for the counselor, therefore, is to provide a therapeutic situation in which a young child is engaged, active and comfortable enough within the activity to allow the family drama to unfold in such a way that real learning, growth and change can take place.

When planning experiential activities for families with young children, the counselor needs to consider the special needs of children in a variety of areas. These include: (a) program orientation, (b) attention ability, (c) physical and verbal skills, d) involvement in multi-family interactions, e) cultural background, and (f) special challenges. These topics are discussed in this chapter.

Orientation

A child must be as thoroughly oriented to the nature of the experiential activities as is every other family member. This means explaining, in a child's terms, what is likely to happen. The counselor should be warmly supportive, matter-of-fact and positive, and should avoid wordy explanations that might confuse a child or create apprehension. Descriptions should be exceptionally concrete, even to the point of previewing with a child an outdoor field, gym, classroom, or other areas where activities are likely to take place. Environment is important to young children (Markowitz, 1997), and a particular child's response to a room, outdoor field, weather conditions, and other environmental factors should be taken into consideration in planning.

A child should also be encouraged to look at and handle some of the materials such as balls, ropes, wooden blocks, art materials, etc., which will be used in the program. Items that are distressing to the child for any reason should be eliminated. This time gives the counselor the opportunity to assess the child's activity level, verbal and physical skills, personality, emotional response, listening and communication skills, sociability, and level of cooperation. The child has the opportunity to reduce his or her fear of the unknown, ask questions, and begin to build a sense of trust in the counselor.

The child will also unconsciously store away some very important metalevel information leading to the conclusion, "It's okay to be here." The counselor's calm manner, pleasant tone of voice, respectful communication, patience, and sensitivity to the child's concerns will contribute to the child's positive anticipation of the process ahead.

Following a well-crafted orientation, the counselor can begin to develop a plan for therapy with a realistic knowledge of the child. This will help avoid major adjustments during the experiential activities which would be distracting for everyone.

Attention Span

Though attention span typically increases with a child's age, the counselor should not make assumptions about a child's ability to attend to instructions, follow directions, or stay tuned-in to an activity. A child's attentiveness during the orientation will provide some guidelines for planning, but a child's attention span will fluctuate depending on the type of activity, her or his comfort level with other participants, level of hunger or fatigue, distractibility to the environment, and interest level. Activities should be planned with contingencies for what will be done if the child is unable to be attentive.

Physical and Verbal Skills

We know that developmental age and developmental level often do not correspond to established norms in some children (Winnicott, 1965). The counselor should not make assumptions based on chronology. What is this particular child capable of at this particular time? Activities that require skills way beyond a child's ability to perform will cause a great deal of frustration for everyone in the family. The counselor should be willing and able to adapt an activity at any point in order to help keep the experience useful.

On the other hand, it should be up to the family members to find ways to accomplish goals while taking a child's physical and verbal skills into consideration. Counselors need to be careful to not jump in too quickly to save the family from facing a problem in the experiential therapy process. Problem-solving skills related to young children can be weak in some families, and family members may not get a clear picture of how they function unless they are faced with a dramatization of their approach.

There should also be no set standard for good performance. If a certain task is assigned to the family, such as climbing a wall, crossing a "pit," or making a collage, the family should feel free to be flexible with one another in completing the task in such a way that the child and other family members feel a sense of support and accomplishment. A family should never feel the counselor is measuring them against any benchmark, or that there is any preconceived right or wrong way to reach a goal.

Multi-family Groups

When several families with young children are grouped together in an experiential program format, the counselor has to attend not only to the issues being raised within individual families, but also to the interplay between various families. The crucial factor in helping these sessions go well is having enough staff to work with the families, on a one-to-one basis, if necessary, to problem-solve issues as they arise. Counselors should be resources for these families, stepping in when necessary to help them stay on track, deal with intense feelings, or to help with children who begin acting out. Sometimes one angry, frustrated child can start a chain reaction, and an entire multifamily activity falls apart. Counselors may need to stop the action, help the participants deal with the issues, and assist them in moving forward.

Competition, whether planned or spontaneous, can cause individual families to get stuck as they attempt to compete with the other families. A child who is pressured to perform may actively rebel, or the child's participation may become overlooked or minimized in favor of the family "winning." In these situations, when winning becomes the primary goal, a child's need to participate or to have a sense of accomplishment may be preempted by the family's need to win. Children who become extremely frustrated by this usually find a way to communicate it, often through angry outbursts, fighting with siblings, attacking a parent, or simply collapsing on the floor or ground in tears. In these situations it is not uncommon for a family to simply stop participating and not know how to continue. Counselors must be prepared to process the situation on the spot, as needed, and help the family evaluate specific behaviors, problem-solving strategies and values later during the multi-family processing session.

Cultural Issues

Expectations of children vary considerably among different cultures. It is extremely important to remember that, in the absence of abuse in any form, behavior is only a problem if the family considers it a problem. Counselors must plan activities which respect and support a family's cultural beliefs.

It is unethical and destructive to encourage behaviors that threaten a family's cultural value system, regardless of how different the counselor's own belief system may be. The counselor must continually evaluate the extent to which her own personal values influence the types of interventions selected or the manner in which they are processed, especially when the counselor and the family are from two different cultures.

The obvious exception is when it is clear that someone in the family is being harmed. Even then, except in cases where mandated reporter issues are evident, care must be taken to maintain rapport with family members while the concern is being addressed. This is a highly sensitive area for both counselors and families. Counselors should not hesitate to seek supervision or advice from colleagues, if needed.

Challenged Children

A family living and functioning together is a family, regardless of the characteristics of its members. Children with developmental disabilities, sight or hearing impairments, physical, emotional or intellectual challenges have varying levels of capabilities and strengths. None of these characteristics disqualify the children from participating in the experiential activities. Interventions must be individualized carefully to fit family needs.

Again, the orientation phase of planning should provide the counselor with enough information to plan groups which take every family member's needs into consideration. Any family which understands the theory and practice of experiential counseling and is willing and motivated to participate can benefit from an experiential program, provided the counselor is skilled in planning for the family's special needs.

Summary

When asked to describe some of their more memorable counseling situations, many experiential family counselors relate things that young children have said or done. When allowed and encouraged to express themselves freely without fear of criticism, emotional or physical abuse, and when treated with respect, children have a way of getting to the heart of the matter of family issues. They have amazing intuitive strength and often make comments and statements that are purely honest, uncalculated, amazingly accurate, and many times, clever and funny. They add special dimensions of openness and guilelessness that are much harder to reach in families of well-defended adults and older children. It is a serious mistake to assume that young children will play an insignificant role in experiential-based programs. Underestimating their wisdom is a disservice to everyone involved.

On the other hand, overestimating children sets them up to fail. If they do not recognize that the expectations for them are too high, they may try to reach these expectations and be unable to succeed. If they clearly see that they cannot do what is being asked, children may refuse to try, which also feels like failure to them.

Counselors who bring as few preconceived ideas about young children as possible into their assessment and planning activities will avoid misjudging a particular child's capabilities.

When the participation of young children is welcomed, planned for, and carefully managed, experiential activities can address problem issues that reflect real-life family dynamics. As children and other family members together act out the interconnectedness of their roles, problems and solutions become apparent and manageable. By their lack of sophistication and defenses and their willingness to speak honestly, young children often add a special dimension to the counseling process.

Experiential Family Counseling with Adolescents

Stephanie Bryson, LISW

When conjuring an image of more traditional family therapy, one might picture a petulant 13-year-old girl "mad-dogging" her mother or a slouching, baggy-clothed 16-year-old male on the corner of the couch. Given the difficulties families often face during this challenging life cycle stage, the likelihood of seeing an adolescent in family therapy is high. The presenting problem is often an issue of separation-individuation, as the family system tries to restructure rules and limits to accommodate the adolescent member's need for increased autonomy and independence (Garcia-Preto, 1989).

Developmental Issues in Family Therapy with Adolescents

This need for the adolescent's greater autonomy and independence often serves as a catalyst in the family system, putting pressure on the family's structure and sometimes invoking change among at least three generations. The family system's job—to support its adolescent members in making good life choices in the fast-paced, technologically saturated, globally capitalist world of the 21st century—has become increasingly difficult. Parents (guardians or grandparents) are often at a loss to understand why their children are behaving as they are. They may have difficulty understanding just how complicated their adolescent's world has become.

Parents may also experience fear of loss, grief, and rejection as their teens present them with requests for greater freedom and as the children who were sweet as ten-year-olds undergo physical, sexual, and identity changes. Parents may especially feel this way if they experienced abandonment in their own adolescence. So how can experiential family therapy be useful to all of its members, adolescent and others when the needs and wants of the members may differ substantially?

Experiential Family Counseling with Adolescents

When one thinks about experiential or wilderness programming, adolescents readily come to mind—a psychiatric inpatient group of kids helping each other scale a 20-foot wall, a community group untangling a human knot, former gang members painting a mural. Group experiential therapy and group activities generally make sense for a peer-oriented developmental cohort. Teens need to learn in groups so they can master the complicated developmental tasks of adolescence.

Adolescents are often the most dynamic, enthusiastic participants in an experiential family activity. Adolescents in this type of counseling can serve as untapped reservoirs of deep insight into the family system's intergenerational conflicts. When asked, adolescents will say that what they want is for their parents to notice them, support them, set some rules, and give them more freedom—without a battle. Teens generally want to remain connected with family members but don't know how to accomplish the tasks of separation and individuation without adopting certain disrespectful attitudes or becoming irritable and hostile when they feel judged. The following guidelines can assist the practitioner in working successfully with adolescents in experiential family counseling.

Providing Opportunities for Leadership

Adolescents can be an underutilized source of leadership potential in family experiential exercises. The success of experiential work rests, in part, on the practitioner's ability to communicate respect for an adolescent's ability to provide leadership during the session.

Adolescents can be recruited into helping with an experiential exercise. Rarely is an adolescent unwilling to help the clinician. More often, they are relieved to have a focus which diverts them from the sometimes excruciating process of having the counseling examine their shortcomings. The clinician can appeal to an adolescent's willingness to help, to be recognized as an important member of the family, and to the adolescent's desire to attract the ever-elusive positive attention so often mentioned in traditional family therapy settings. Examples include asking the adolescent to help set up some of the props needed for a particular activity or eliciting from him information about how he would approach a particular problem presented in an exercise.

Of course, the clinician should assess the family and the particular adolescent before proceeding in this way. Some adolescents—particularly shy, depressed, or extremely disturbed kids—may feel put on the spot and made unnecessarily anxious. The clinician must also assess the cultural appropriateness of the activity and of the adolescent's willingness to help.

By taking such a stance, the clinician communicates, through actions, that the teen's opinion and work will be valued in this setting. Parents also will get the opportunity to observe their son or daughter interacting with another adult, something they may not have much occasion to do.

Although it is desirable to ally with the adolescent in the family system, the practitioner must be very careful not to over-ally with her, a common mistake of clinicians whose own adolescent and self-image issues get activated. Although adolescents may pull for a peer relationship with the clinician, the clinician must bear in mind that ultimately, trying to be friends with an adolescent member of a family group is contraindicated. The clinician will often be in the position of modeling the complex relationship a parent needs to have with daughter or son during this process, an adult-child relationship based on respect and clear, appropriate boundaries as well as positive encouragement.

Positive Communication

Positive communication is the elixir of success when working with adolescents. Their self-esteem and moods fluctuate a great deal based on their perception of their likableness, their talents, and their popularity with their peers. While adolescents certainly need guidance, they need it to be tailored to their fluctuations. Adolescents, in particular, need accurate feedback about their positive qualities, efforts, and accomplishments during an activity. Of course, the clinician will want to elicit as much of this as possible from the parents or other family members. An adolescent should never be spared positive feedback because it is an essential component of successful identity formation. As teens are consistently and accurately recognized in different settings and relationships, they begin to form a stable, core identity that will accompany them into their next developmental challenge. Adolescents, fragile as they sometimes seem, can hear and tolerate a surprising amount of constructive criticism if it is preceded by accurate positive feedback.

Since adolescents are often strong group members during the exercises, there are ample opportunities for giving them positive feedback. The processing or debriefing sessions that typically follow the experiential exercises are a great time to provide such feedback.

Power Struggles and Resistance

Power struggles between adolescents and parents are chief among presenting problems in family therapy settings. Adolescents are working very hard to learn to exert some amount of control over their complicated lives. They will have to manage their lives in a few years and are trying, in earnest, to figure out how to do all the things they are asked to master during this developmental period. They, understandably, are concerned with gracefully pulling off this huge developmental task. In most families, teens face a number of expectations from family and extended family members. They don't want to lose face. They want to feel good about themselves, to experience themselves as competent and worthy. And they need to develop a sense of purpose, power, and efficacy (Brendtro, Brokenleg, & Van Bockern, 1990).

In experiential settings, the distribution of power is one of the dynamics that can be most readily identified by the clinician and, in some exercises, modified or controlled. If an adolescent is unwilling to participate, the clinician must first try to understand why. Does the environment feel safe enough? Is the adolescent holding a big family secret? Is she shy? Is she worried she will be uncoordinated? Is she worried she will be ridiculed by another family member? If an adolescent is simply seeming ornery, the clinician might want to focus on a role which will elicit mastery, competence, and power. One might try to give an unwilling adolescent an important observing role to draw them into the activity. Just as with younger children, adolescents do well when given at least some choices rather than an edict. A resistant or quiet adolescent may be the key to unlocking very important family dynamics.

Gender and Sexual Orientation

Bearing in mind the difficulty of adolescent identity development, the practitioner should take care not to assume that the adolescent is dating or sexually active or is not seriously considering or involved in a relationship with a member of the same gender. Gay and lesbian teens, like teens from other marginalized identity groups, suffer a great deal of harassment from their families and peers. They comprise a disproportionate number of teen suicides committed every year. Clinicians should take care to use gender nonspecific pronouns in all their discussions with family if they wish to ensure maximum safety and participation from teens who are dealing with sexual orientation issues.

Gay and lesbian adolescents will often test the clinician in subtle ways to ascertain whether he or she is a safe, knowledgeable adult. They will often put out extremely sensitive antennae to check the clinician out. As stated in the first section of this book, experiential exercises elicit a more genuine and less guarded exposure of the client's personality. In this type of setting, they may want to disclose their sexual orientation. Sometimes, adolescents are hoping the clinician will assist them in telling their family. Other times, the teen simply wants to be seen accurately by a nonjudgemental, accepting adult.

Art & Music

Adolescents almost always enjoy family experiential exercises involving art or music. If an adolescent is difficult to engage, these are two areas that often yield success. The adolescent, if refusing to participate in an activity, can be asked to draw the event as other family members take part. Similarly, the adolescent can be asked to bring in music they like for certain activities. Inviting these two adolescent-friendly areas into the family counseling can yield surprising results.

Humor

Although most practitioners of experiential family counseling come to the work with a good sense of humor, it never hurts to remember what a powerful medium humor can be with all members of a family. Adolescents seem to respond to respectful, appropriate humor used by a clinician. The fun, playful nature of the experiential exercises lends itself to the use of humor. Confident clinicians can use goofy, light-hearted self-reproach or calculated self-disclosure to point out human frailties and thus normalize all human behavior.

Guiding Metaphor and Summary

It is helpful for clinicians from all fields and modalities to keep in mind some guiding principles about the developmental challenges of adolescence. Adolescence requires that the young adult have a stable, dependable adult and a safe-enough holding environment from which to launch his or her explorations of the world. Goodness-of-fit is important for optimum developmental progress in adolescence. If adults are too protective with a gregarious teen, or if they are unresponsive to a more sensitive adolescent temperament, goodness-of-fit is compromised and, with it, the tasks of identity formation and separation-individuation. The clinician needs to continually assess the goodness-of-fit between the adolescent and the experiential activities and adjust them accordingly. This needs to be done at the same time as assessing the other family members' needs and also modifying the exercises to match the needs—quite a task!

Although they may ask to be treated as adults, and sometimes induce adults to behave like children, adolescents are searching for adults who can model being adults— self-assured, flexible, warm, compassionate, competent adults who neither capitulate to childish behavior nor enshrine themselves in the defended adult world of insecurity and arrogance. Adolescents seek out the real thing in adults and can help us grow as clinicians when we commit to behave in the best interest of our young adult clients.

The Counseling Session

The section describes the actual experiential counseling session. An outline of a suggested counseling session structure follows:

- ☐ Introduction/Review the Purpose and Goals of Counseling
- ☐ Physical and Emotional Check-In
- ☐ Statement of Participant Rights and Responsibilities
- ☐ Name Game (if needed)
- ☐ Contracting (if needed)
- ☐ Warm-Ups
- ☐ The Family Problem-Solving Initiative(s)
- ☐ Session Debrief and Review
- ☐ Closure

Introduction/ Review Program Goals

Even if a thorough program orientation has been conducted, the first session should include a brief introduction to the program. It is often effective to tell a few short stories about other families who have participated in the program (not using names or identifying features to protect confidentiality). This might include also describing what they have said about the program, or telling a personal story about a particular activity or event.

All subsequent sessions begin with family participants describing, in a "go-around-the-circle" format, one special learning that stands out from the previous session. This introductory time can also be used to clarify the purpose and goals of the particular session.

Physical and Emotional Safety Check

Although the family activities are not inherently dangerous, experiential-based activities often involve some physical and psychological risks. General and specific safety policies need to be established which enable the participants to minimize those hazards associated with risk-taking. The counseling goals of the program can best be achieved through voluntary participation in perceived risk activities within a safe, trusting, and supportive atmosphere. Individuals are encouraged to participate fully and openly, but not carelessly. Program facilitators and the participants are to view safety as their main concern and the most influential guide in all aspects of the program.

PEEP is a helpful acronym used to facilitate the safety discussion at the beginning of each family session. The PEEP check assists the counselor in setting a climate of physical and emotional safety. The acronym stands for Physical Check, Emotional Check, Environmental Check, and Personal Check.

The PEEP check or any component of it can also be used during the counseling sessions at a time when the counselor or any participant thinks there is a safety issue. Participants should be encouraged to take charge of their own physical and psychological safety by making others aware when they feel their own or another group member's safety is in jeopardy. Following is a discussion of the principles of the PEEP safety check.

PEEP: The Creation of Safe Space as a Norm in Experiential Family Counseling

by Juli Lynch

Introduction

When using experiential counseling activities, the counselor is an expert, not only in the technical aspects, but also in the interpersonal aspects of the experience. By providing a framework and boundaries, the counselor allows for a safe space to be established, a space in which families can focus their attention and energy on the therapy instead of on threats to their emotional or physical well-being.

The counselor provides a definition of the boundaries for the counseling session. If these boundaries are explicit and the behaviors implying the boundaries are reinforced, a safe space can be offered as a norm in the life of the counseling group.

Safety procedures, the rationale behind the procedures, the instructions given about them, and the reinforcement of the procedures influence the adoption of the safety-related behavioral norms. These norms, once established, influence the process of the experience and in some respect govern whether the family has a safe or unsafe experience. Deviations from the norm can create potential compromises to safety.

The PEEP Safety Check

One technique that explicitly outlines the behaviors required to ensure safety among family participants in an experiential counseling setting is PEEP. PEEP represents: Physical, Emotional, Environmental and Personal safety.

The purpose of PEEP is to provide a framework of emotional and physical safety for the counseling session. PEEP assumes that the counselor takes the initial stance as the expert in physical and emotional safety with the intention of facilitating the family towards becoming the experts.

PEEP assumes that a climate of emotional and physical safety is most conducive to meaningful learning. Within a safe space, risk-taking is more likely to occur. For the family, PEEP offers a defined framework within which the experience will occur. Initial anxiety about the session is relieved when families are given clear, concise and concrete information on procedures for maintaining not only their physical safety but also their emotional safety.

Framework

"Safety is the number one priority" is stated with an emphasis on emotional as well as physical safety of all family members.

P–Physical

States that the family and the counselor need to know of the group's physical concerns. Another goal of the Physical check is to demonstrate that the family is in charge of letting one another know of any physical concerns that come up during or after the experience or both.

E–Emotional

Requests that families begin by sharing their here and now feelings. The guidelines of the Emotional check include:

- Family members volunteer to speak only for themselves and not for other members.
- Family members avoid sarcasm as a way to communicate. They are asked to practice direct expression of feelings.
- Family members practice supportive styles of communication.
- Family members allow each family member to choose her or his level of involvement.

E–Environmental

States that the family and the counselor are in charge of keeping one another aware of any potential environmental hazards (equipment, weather, rocks, sticks, chairs, tables, etc.)

P–Personal

States that all jewelry that can hurt oneself or another must be removed—rings, watches, necklaces. No gum chewing, cigarette smoking, eating or drinking is allowed during the counseling session. Proper clothing and footwear are encouraged.

Stop Mechanism

States that, at any point during the experience, any member, either a family member or the counselor, has the absolute right and the absolute responsibility to call a PEEP Check or a time out. At the moment a PEEP is called, all activity is stopped (within reason) and the safety issue is addressed. The assumption is that if any member perceives an unsafe situation, it must be acknowledged. Because safety is the number one priority, the safety concern must be addressed and resolved to the satisfaction of all participants.

Methodology

The counselor begins the counseling session by asking the family to form a circle. This positions the family neutrally and aligns the counselor alongside the family. The counselor begins by stating, "The number one priority of the session is safety." The counselor may engage the family in a discussion about why safety is so important. Usually families initially focus on physical aspects of safety. The counselor can also introduce the concept of emotional safety and engage the family in a discussion on its meaning.

The counselor then states that during the program sessions, PEEP will be used to assist everyone in remembering guidelines for safety. PEEP is introduced clearly and concisely, including all of the points mentioned above. In the initial session the explanation of PEEP may take up a fair amount of time. It is important that the family acquires this knowledge in order to begin the process of "normalizing " PEEP into the program.

The explanation is concluded with a verbal description of the "Stop" mechanism. It is stressed that the counselor as well as family members can call a safety check anytime they feel as though the emotional or physical safety of any family member is in jeopardy. It is made clear that a safety check can be called for oneself or for another member. It is further explained that when one is called, all action will stop and the family along with the counselor will focus on the concern to find a solution to eliminate the unsafe situation.

After the introduction and explanation of PEEP, the counselor leads the family through a PEEP check. For the first P, Physical, family members as well as the counselor in a round-the-circle format verbalize any physical concerns (bad back, sore knee, asthma, stomachache, etc.).

For the first E, Emotional, a feeling check is done in a round-the-circle manner for check-ins. Check-ins can be utilized by the counselor or the family members to clarify feeling statements made by any member. The counselor should establish a norm of checking-in when family members state feelings which are vague or have negative connotations. The counselor can model the behavior by asking the family member if they think they can stay safe, despite those feelings, during the family session.

Next, the counselor asks the family to identify the second E, Environmental concerns. Here the family should observe their physical surrounding and identify conditions that could potentially cause an injury or create an accident.

For the second P, Personal, a PEEP bucket or bag for valuables can be placed in the center of the circle. After "body checks" are made, each participant states clearly that he or she is safe in a round-the-circle check. The last part of the PEEP check should include a verbal reminder of the Stop mechanism and the expectation and right of each family member and the counselor to use it.

Normalizing

The counselor should normalize the use of PEEP safety checks by calling them as they occur during the session. In addition, the counselor can verbally reinforce the calling of PEEPs by other family members.

The counselor should work towards transferring ownership of PEEP to the family. This is done in subsequent sessions by having the family open the session by initiating their own PEEP check.

PEEP as an Intervention

In the initial session PEEP can be an intervention that alleviates much of the initial anxiety that is brought by a family into an experiential-based setting. Its concrete guidelines provide an anchoring point and structure for families who often have minimal structure.

It also offers the counselor an opportunity to provide a psycho education intervention. Often, the family struggles with a lack of resources for incorporating the Emotional boundaries of PEEP. The counselor can use PEEP and its guidelines in the context of an experiential exercise to teach skills of communication, conflict resolution, and respect for personal and physical space.

PEEP also can be used as an intervention in teaching families to care for themselves as individuals and as a family unit. The Stop mechanism as an intervention reinforces the creation of a safe space for family development and enhancement. For example, when brother expresses his anger by being overly aggressive toward sister, mom can call a safety check and express her concern that neither sister nor brother are behaving in a safe manner. Or during an argument between mom and dad, a daughter can call a safety check to express her own lack of emotional safety when hearing and witnessing the fighting.

One of the unexpected, yet reasonable outgrowths of the use of PEEP has been the adoption by families of a model similar to PEEP as a norm outside of the counseling sessions. A number of families report that this has become an integral guideline for monitoring safe emotional and physical behavior within the home.

Summary

In experiential-based counseling, counselors have an ethical responsibility to provide safe experiences for their clients. Counselors have the responsibility of not only establishing technical safety, but also promoting the emotional safety of their clients. PEEP can be tossed into a counselor's bag of tricks to be utilized as psychological safety equipment.

The PEEP Safety Checklist

_____ Physical Check

A physical check is conducted to identify any bumps, bruises, injuries (past or present), medical conditions, and level of "alertness-tiredness" that may affect an individual's or the group's performance. A "go-round", with each participant having an opportunity to respond, is used to give each individual an opportunity to discuss any physical limitations.

_____ Emotional Check

An emotional or feelings check is also conducted as a go-round-the-circle with participants having an opportunity to describe their emotional state. Each participant chooses one or two words to describe how he or she is feeling at the present moment. Following the "go-round", the counselor or another participant can check-in with any participant, asking that participant to describe his or her feelings in further detail. This check helps to insure that the participants are emotionally prepared for the counseling session.

_____ Environmental Check

The participants are asked to take further responsibility for their safety by identifying all those elements in their immediate physical environment that may have the potential to cause injury or harm (e.g., obstacles, furniture, weather hazards, uneven ground, etc.).

_____ Personal Check

This step asks participants to remove all jewelry, items in pockets, large belt buckles, or any other personal items that can cause injury to self and others. This procedure is used when the exercises involve physical activity.

Experiential Check-In Activities

The purpose of the check-in activities is to assist the counselor and family members in setting a climate of psychological safety. This check helps to ensure that the participants are emotionally prepared for the counseling session. Because children and youth are often activity-driven, experiential-based exercises are often more effective as check-in tools. The following five experiential activities offer alternatives to a verbal check-in.

Movement Chain

Goal

Each family member uses a group movement game to describe his or her current emotional state.

Materials Required

25' section of rope with ends tied to make a circle.

Procedures

All family members grab a piece of the rope circle. One member of the group begins making a movement, using the rope to describe how he or she is currently feeling. Ask all other members to mimic that movement so that a group movement with the rope results. Past examples have included a vigorous bicycle-pedal movement with the rope between hands to represent stress and a rocking of the rope from side to side above heads to symbolize excitement. Give each person an opportunity to use this method to describe how he or she is currently feeling.

Variation

Each person gets an opportunity to give instructions to the other family members (who are holding a section of the rope circle) to create a shape with the rope that represents that person's most prevalent feeling at the present time. For example, a family member may ask the group to make a square using the rope because he is feelings a bit edgy.

Musical Feelings

Goal

Family members use musical instruments to express their emotional state.

Materials Required

An assortment of toy musical instruments (those often found in elementary school classes)

Procedures

Give participants an opportunity to freely explore the sounds of various instruments. Then, ask members to take turns selecting a musical instrument and creating a sound (stressing tempo and loudness) that best expresses how she is feeling at the present time.

Biblio Check-In

Goal

Family members express how they are feeling through referencing a story.

Materials Required

One of the following books:

a. *Quick as a Cricket* by Audrey Wood (This is a book of personal descriptors—e.g., "I am as busy as a bee," "I'm as quiet as a lark," "I'm as gentle as a lamb," "I'm as mean as a shark," etc.), or

b. *My Many Colored Days* by Dr. Suess (This book describes feelings as colors—e.g., "Some days are brown and I feel low, low down;" "Some days are gray, nothing moves today."

Procedures

As the chosen book is read aloud to the group, instruct the participants to think about which page is most like him or her at the present time. Then, in a round-the-group fashion, give each person an opportunity to pick the page and show the rest of the group their selected descriptor page.

Puppet Check-In

Goal

Family members use a puppet to describe their feelings at the present time.

Materials Required

- ☐ An assortment of puppets (Inexpensive sets can be purchased from school supply catalogs), or
- ☐ Brown paper lunch bags and markers can be used by participants to create their own puppets.

Procedures

Give each person an opportunity to select or create a puppet. Ask them to let the puppet "friend" tell the rest of the group how her or his human friend is feeling today.

Pick A Feeling

Goal

Family members use visual feeling "cards" to express how they are feeling.

Materials Required

Visual representations of feelings—e.g. feeling charts, feeling expressions drawn on cards, different types of feeling faces drawn on paper plates, etc.

Procedures

Give each person, in a go-around-the-group exercise, the opportunity to select the visual symbol that best expresses how she or he is feeling.

Participant Rights and Responsibilities

Goals: The goals of the Participant Rights and Responsibilities are:

☐ to set a climate of emotional safety, and
☐ to relieve tension.

Procedure

At the beginning of each session, following the check-in, each participant is given a copy of the Participant Rights and Responsibilities (see following pages). The counselor introduces this exercise by stating that it is really important that all members understand their rights before they start the session.

The rights are read as a go-round with each person taking a turn reading a right in the order of their listing. Because one of the rights is "the right to remain silent or 'pass' during group discussions," members are told that for whatever reason, they may pass and do not have to read a right. This protects those individuals, both children and adults, who have difficulty with reading.

The counselor ensures that all group members understand each of the rights. For example, the first right uses the word confidentiality. The counselor may want to ask someone in the group to define this word.

A way to continue developing a climate of safety based on personal rights is to ask each member to choose the Participant Right that is most important to him or her at the present time. Each member is given the opportunity to share with the rest of the group the right she or he selected. Not only does this give each participant an indirect, nonthreatening way to voice needs, it also provides the counselor with assessment information as to those concerns that are most relevant to the participants. For example, a mother may state that the right that stands out most for her is "the right to be heard and taken seriously." This may be an indication to both the counselor and her family that she may feel unheard in her family.

After the Participant Bill of Rights are read, the Participant Responsibilities are read in the same manner. The counselor also encourages the group to call a safety check (as described in PEEP) at any time during any situation in which they believe the Rights and Responsibilities are not being followed.

Participant Bill of Rights

- ☐ I have the right to confidentiality and privacy by the staff and other group and family members.
- ☐ I have the right to remain silent or "pass" during group discussions.
- ☐ I have the right to choose to participate or not participate in any of the activities or discussions.
- ☐ I have the right to be treated with respect by the other family and group members.
- ☐ I have the right to ask for and receive physical and emotional support from the other family and group members.
- ☐ I have the right to express my feelings, thoughts and opinions.
- ☐ I have the right to be listened to and taken seriously.
- ☐ I have the right to make mistakes.
- ☐ I have the right to celebrate personal and family successes.
- ☐ I have the right to say, "I don't understand."
- ☐ I have the right to say, "No!"
- ☐ I have the right to decide how and who will enter into my personal space.
- ☐ I have the right NOT to have the values of others forced on me.
- ☐ I have the right NOT to be exposed to excess pressure from the other family and group members.

Participant Responsibilities

- [ ] I will preserve confidentiality by respecting the privacy of the other group and family members.
- [ ] I will participate in program activities and exercises at a level which I still believe is my choice.
- [ ] I will speak only for myself and not for other family and group members.
- [ ] I will ask for what I want and need.
- [ ] I will be willing to take risks.
- [ ] I will be willing to talk about myself.
- [ ] I will treat the other group and family members with respect, even when I don't agree with their behavior or viewpoints.
- [ ] I will express feelings in ways that show respect for the dignity of the other group and family members.

Contracts

A contract, as defined for this program, is a written agreement between family members stating desirable behavior for the counseling session. Contracts assist with identifying and clearly stating those behaviors that will facilitate a positive and growth-producing experience for all of the family participants.

Two types of contracts are presented:

- ☐ *The Family Contract* can aid all types of families in setting healthy guidelines for their counseling experience.
- ☐ *The Behavioral Contract* can be used for families with children or adolescents who have some difficulties controlling their impulsive and inappropriate behaviors and need a tool to assist with some additional structures.

These two contracts are further described on the following pages.

The Family Contract:

The family contract is a simple, norm-setting tool that can be used with all families. It asks families to specify the behaviors that they will use to make the session or program a positive experience for each other and for the other families. An example of The Family Contract can be found on the following page.

The Family Contract

Task

To create a family contract, through consensus, which states those standards of behavior your family will use to develop a supportive environment during your family program, an environment where personal and family goals are most likely to be achieved.

Procedure

In family groups, family members brainstorm those behaviors and attitudes that will assist each family member, the family unit, and the other family groups in having a positive experience. In other words, the contract should address the following questions:

a. What can we do as a family to ensure that each of our family members has a positive experience?

b. What can we do as a family unit to assist in developing a climate in which the other families and family members have a positive experience?

The Family Contract

We, the members of this family, agree on the date of ___/___/__ to use and practice the following behaviors and attitudes during our period of involvement in the family program:

1.

2.

3.

4.

Use back side of this paper, if necessary.

The Behavioral Contract

The Behavioral Contract is used for families with children or young adolescents when their behaviors can be or have been a problem during the program. The behavioral contract is a systematic procedure for establishing agreements between parents and their children for the purpose of behavioral change. These written contracts explicitly describe agreements and specify the means, rewards, and consequences of fulfilling the contract. "The written contracts delineate desired behaviors to be rewarded and encourage family members to assign value to specific behaviors and consequences" (Fatis & Konewko, 1983, p. 161).

An example of the Behavioral Contract can be found on the following pages.

The general steps are:

1. Identify those behaviors that are problematic or can be potentially problematic during the program activities. The Acceptable/Unacceptable Behaviors form may be used for this purpose.
2. Establish behavioral standards, rewards for maintenance, and consequences for noncompliance, which can be achieved by employing the Behavioral Family Contract.

Acceptable/Unacceptable Behaviors Form

Directions: Please complete this worksheet by indicating the level of acceptability of the following behaviors by your family members during the program activities. Work as a family to decide what is acceptable and what is unacceptable. Circle the appropriate number.

	Acceptable Behavior		Moderately Unacceptable Behavior		Totally Unacceptable Behavior
not listening	1	2	3	4	5
speaking when someone else is speaking	1	2	3	4	5
not following directions	1	2	3	4	5
withdrawing/pouting	1	2	3	4	5
refusing to try activities	1	2	3	4	5
giving up	1	2	3	4	5
not respecting the personal space of others	1	2	3	4	5
arguing/fighting with other family members	1	2	3	4	5
physically fighting with others	1	2	3	4	5
being disruptive by demanding attention	1	2	3	4	5
using insults and vulgar language/gestures	1	2	3	4	5
not following parents' directions	1	2	3	4	5

Behavioral Family Contract

Directions: The child and parent(s) are to work together to negotiate standards of acceptable behaviors of the child during the family program. The reward for fulfilling the contract and the consequence for not fulfilling the contract are also to be negotiated.

A. Standard of Acceptable Behavior:

Reward for Maintaining the Standard:

Consequence if Acceptable Behavior is Not Maintained:

B. Standard of Acceptable Behavior:

Reward for Maintaining the Standard:

Consequence if Acceptable Behavior is Not Maintained:

For the Parent:

I (We),_____, the parent(s) of _____, on the date of ___/___/___, agree to provide my son/daughter with the support and assistance to allow him/her to fulfill this contract. I also agree to consistently implement the rewards and consequences as specified in this contract.

Signature of Parent(s): _____

To the Child:

I,_____, on the date of ___/___/___, agree to maintain and practice the standards of acceptable behavior as specified in this contract to the best of my ability. I also agree to readily accept those rewards and consequences specified in this contract.

Signature of Child: _____

A Sample Behavioral Family Contract

Directions: The child and parent(s) work together to negotiate standards of acceptable behaviors for the child during the family program including rewards for following the behavior and consequences for not maintaining that standard.

A. Standard of Acceptable Behavior:

Johnny is to keep quiet and listen when another family or group member is speaking.

Reward for Maintaining the Standard:

Johnny will be complemented by his parents.

Consequence if Acceptable Behavior is Not Maintained

Johnny will be asked to step out of the group until he makes a commitment to the group that he is ready to listen to and respect others.

B. Standard of Acceptable Behavior:

Johnny is to respect the rights of his younger sister by not screaming at her, insulting her, using vulgar language around her, or hitting her.

Reward for Maintaining the Standard:

Johnny can earn extra money ($3 per family session) to be used on a special family outing.

Consequence if Acceptable Behavior is Not Maintained:

Johnny will be: 1) given an initial warning, 2) given a second warning, 3) given a ten minute time out.

Name Games and Warm-Ups

Purpose

Name Games and Warm-Ups assist participants in becoming familiar with the program format and the personality styles of the counselor and other family groups. Name games and warm-ups help alleviate tensions and anxieties associated with being placed in an unfamiliar situation, and they set a tone for the experience.

Strategies

- ☐ Choose Warm-Ups that elicit the active involvement of all participants.
- ☐ Select Warm-Ups to meet the characteristics of the participating group's culture:

  a. What types of Warm-Ups will be acceptable for that group? Will they be too silly or too embarrassing?
  b. Can they produce feelings of failure? If so, others should be selected.
  c. Will the Warm-Ups match the mental, emotional, and physical characteristics of the group?
  d. Will they be acceptable given the cultural norms of the group?

- ☐ Relate Warm-Ups to the overall program goals.
- ☐ Keep Warm-Ups dynamic and fast moving. Specific Warm-Ups should be discontinued if hints of boredom are observed.

Sample Name Games and Warm-Ups are found on the following pages.

Name Games

When working with in a multifamily group format, participants often do not know the names of the members from other families. One of the first tasks of the counselor is to facilitate the learning of each other's names. When sessions are spread out over several weeks, name games may be needed every session.

Toss a Name

Materials Required

Several small balls.

Procedure

1. Ask the group to stand in a circle.
2. Begin by pointing to someone across the circle and asking his or her name. Repeat that person's name while tossing him or her a ball. The catcher responds by saying, "Thank you," and adding the tosser's name. The catcher may have to ask the tosser's name to complete the phrase.
3. This process continues by the catcher becoming the tosser, pointing to someone across the circle, and so forth.
4. For example, Toss a Name may look and sound like: The counselor says, "What is your name?" (while pointing to someone across the circle). The person responds, "Susan." The counselor repeats Susan's name and tosses her the ball. Susan responds to the tosser, "Thank you, what is your name?" The tosser says, "John." Susan says, "Thank you, John." This pattern continues. Susan then points to someone else and asks, "What is your name?" and so on. Additional balls may be added later in the game to increase interest and fun.

Duck, Duck, Goose Name Game

Materials Required

None

Procedure

1. The Duck, Duck, Goose Name Game is a take-off on the childhood game. Ask the group to stand in a tight—almost-shoulder-to-shoulder—circle. One person volunteers to be "It". "It" leaves the circle and his or her "space" in the circle is closed up by the people in the circle.

2. "It" proceeds slowly around the outside circumference of the circle and taps each person on the shoulder while saying "Duck" with each tap. "It" then taps one person's shoulder and says "Goose".

3. The goosed person and "It" walk fast in opposite directions around the outside of the circle. When they cross paths on the opposite side, they stop, shake hands and verbally introduce themselves one at a time, "Hi, my name is _____," and "Hi, my name is _____."

4. After they complete their introduction, they continue walking fast around the circle back to the open spot of the goosed person. The first person back to the spot gets to keep the spot. The last person back becomes "It" and begins the Duck, Duck, Goose Name Game again.

5. Some general guidelines for this game include:

   ☐ You must introduce yourself on your way around. The group can ask you to do it again if they think your introduction was inadequate.
   ☐ Running is not allowed.

The Other Side Of the Blanket

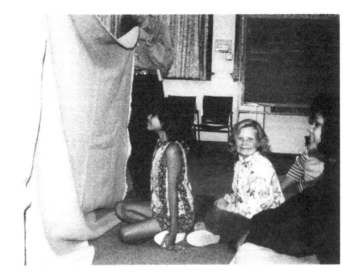

Materials Required

A blanket

Procedure

1. Split the group into two groups, half the participants in one group and the other half in the other group.
2. Encourage participants to learn as many of the names of the members in the other group.
3. Two counselors (or volunteers) hold the blanket up vertically so that it creates a wall between the two groups. One group "hides" behind one side and the other group on the other side (See above). Behind their own side of the blanket, each group secretly picks one of their members to be "It." This person sits in front of the blanket on their side.
4. Once the two group representatives ("Its") are in place, the object becomes for the other team to guess who is "It." One team is chosen to go first. They decide by consensus who from the other side they believe is "It" and then they yell out the name. If their guess is incorrect, the other team yells back "no," and that team is given a chance to make a guess. If their guess is correct, the other team yells, "yes," the blanket is dropped, and the "It" moves over to the team who made the correct guess. The game is played until everyone is on one side or until the game has worn itself out.

Warm-Ups

Family Have You Evers?

Family "Have You Evers" is a fairly nonthreatening warm-up that can be used with any number of family participants or families at any point during the program.

Goals

- ☐ To break the ice and have some fun.
- ☐ To plant some seeds about some fun activities a family can do together.

Materials Required

List of questions for the facilitator

Procedure

Ask the family or families to gather in a large group circle. Read each of the Family "Have You Evers?" (found on the next page). If the family has ever done the thing mentioned, they jump in the middle of the circle and receive a round of applause from themselves, the therapists, and other families. They then move back to the outer circle for the reading of the next item. After the list is completed, the families can be encouraged to make up some of their own items.

"Have You Evers" Questions

Has your family ever . . .

- [ ] been in a pillow fight?
- [ ] been on a picnic?
- [ ] gone camping together?
- [ ] swam in the ocean together?
- [ ] played football together?
- [ ] had a family portrait taken?
- [ ] gone to or sponsored a family reunion?
- [ ] been on a road trip?
- [ ] gone out to dinner together?
- [ ] made up a song together?
- [ ] watched a scary movie together?
- [ ] had a food fight?
- [ ] toasted marshmallows together?
- [ ] been to a mall shopping together?
- [ ] watched a sunset together?
- [ ] been fishing together?
- [ ] baked something together?
- [ ] read stories out loud to one another?
- [ ] done lawn work together?
- [ ] sipped lemonade together on a hot day?
- [ ] played hide and seek together?
- [ ] planted a tree together?
- [ ] climbed a tree together?
- [ ] had tickle "wars?"
- [ ] played a board game together?

Family Scavenger Hunt*

The Family Scavenger Hunt is recommended for multifamily groups and groups in which the family members can read and write, and do this activity with limited supervision.

Goals

- ☐ To have fun and break the ice.
- ☐ To begin the process of self-disclosure.
- ☐ To assist participants of a multifamily group in getting to know one another.

Materials Required

- ☐ One copy of the Family Scavenger Hunt per person (see next page)
- ☐ One pencil or pen per person

Procedures

Distribute the Family Scavenger Hunt work sheets and pencils to the group members. Have them follow the directions given on the sheet.

*Adapted from Weinstein's and Goodman's (1980) Human Treasure Hunt in *Playfair*.

Human Scavenger Hunt

The purpose of this exercise is for you to get better acquainted with your own family as well as with the people from the other families. Find someone from your own family or another family who matches the item. Speak personally to the person. Do not use prior knowledge. Put the appropriate name in the space provided. You should have a different name for each item. Try to contact as many people as possible during this exercise.

Find someone who has laughed out loud with someone from his or her family during the past week. Find out what was funny.

_____

Find two people who view their families as their greatest asset. Discover their most successful family achievements.

_____

Find someone who has and remembers a favorite childhood game. Play that game with him or her.

_____

Find two people who are willing to share their dreams for their family. Have them do some sharing.

_____

Find a person who has a favorite family story. Have him or her tell it to you.

_____

Find someone who has done something unique with his or her family. Find out what it was.

_____

Penny for Your Thoughts

Penny for Your Thoughts is a fairly nonthreatening assessment tool that can be used with any number of family participants or families at any point during the program.

Goals

- ☐ To have fun and break the ice.
- ☐ To begin the process of self-disclosure.
- ☐ To gather personal and assessment data through a fun, nonthreatening activity.

Materials Required

- ☐ Jar of Pennies
- ☐ Question Sheet for the Facilitator

Procedures

1. Ask the family members to sit in a circle with a large pile of pennies in the middle. The family is asked to answer a series of personal questions (see Penny for Your Thoughts Questions sheet on the next page).
2. Ask each family member to answer the question in a round-the-group-circle fashion. They must answer as quickly as possible when it is their turn. If they answer the question, they are allowed to grab one penny from the middle of the circle. If they do not answer the question, if they do not answer the question quickly (within a few seconds of their turn), or if they speak out of turn, they do not receive a penny. The person with the most pennies at the end of the game wins. Note: To make the game fair, questions should begin with a different group member (the next in order) for each consecutive question.

Penny for Your Thoughts Questions

- ☐ How old are you?
- ☐ Where do you live?
- ☐ Where do you work or go to school?
- ☐ How many brothers do you have? sisters?
- ☐ Do you still live with both your parents?
- ☐ What is your favorite food?
- ☐ What is your favorite sport?
- ☐ What is your favorite hobby?
- ☐ What do you want to do when you grow up?
- ☐ What other languages do you speak?
- ☐ What's your favorite movie?
- ☐ What was the last book you read?
- ☐ What's your favorite social activity?
- ☐ What's your favorite arts activity?
- ☐ What is you favorite kind of music?
- ☐ What was your favorite vacation?
- ☐ Who do you most admire in the world?
- ☐ What do you like best about yourself?
- ☐ What one thing would you change about yourself?
- ☐ What one thing would you change about your family?
- ☐ What do you like best about your family?
- ☐ What is the best gift you ever received?
- ☐ What is the best gift you ever gave?
- ☐ If your dad were a cartoon character, who would he be?
- ☐ If your mom were a cartoon character, who would she be?
- ☐ What feeling is easy for you to express?
- ☐ What feeling is hard for you to express?
- ☐ Where is a safe place you typically go?
- ☐ What one thing would you like to be remembered for?

Beach Ball Toss

The Beach Ball Toss asks participants to think abstractly and is, therefore, recommended for older groups.

Goals

- ☐ To break the ice and have some fun.
- ☐ To begin the process of identifying family problems and concerns.
- ☐ To explore how problems are handled and tossed around.

Materials Required

- ☐ One beach ball per two or three people
- ☐ Dry erase fine tip overhead projector pens (washes off)—one per person

Procedures

1. Give a blown-up beach ball and marker pen to each group of two to three people.
2. Ask each group member to write a word or draw a symbol on the beach ball that represents a minor family struggle or concern that they are currently having. Each participant is to take a section of their beach ball to do this task.
3. After they have finished identifying and writing or drawing out their family struggle, give them the task to, as a group, keep all the balls bouncing around in the air.
4. After several minutes, when the group has had enough, end the game.

Follow-Up Questions for the Beach Ball Toss*

After the game has worn itself out, ask the following questions-for-thought. Since this is a warm-up game, participants are asked to ponder the answers as opposed to verbally answering them.

- ☐ Were you initially excited about hitting the balls or did you fear them? How is this similar or dissimilar to the way you typically face your family struggles?
- ☐ During the game, did you want to confront or whack the balls, or did you want to avoid them? Do you want to whack at your family struggles, or do you want to avoid them?
- ☐ Did you need to watch where the ball went after you hit it, or could you just let it go? How is this similar to the way you are coping with your family struggles?
- ☐ When the counselor called a halt to the game, did you want one last whack, or were you happy to end it? How is this similar to how you are feeling about your family struggles?

*Suggested by Dr. Byron Norton

Family Jump Rope

Family Jump Rope has a strong physical component and is recommended for family groups who enjoy physical challenges.

Goals

- ☐ To break the ice and have some fun.
- ☐ To begin the process of building/reinforcing family cooperation.

Materials Required

- ☐ a 20' jump rope

Procedures

1. Give the family the task of making one successful jump, as a family group, of a jump rope that is turned over their heads.
2. The counselor and/or members from another family become the rope-turners, one at either end of the rope. The family participants set themselves up in between the two rope-turners with the rope on one side of them.
3. When the family counts to three, the turners circle the jump rope over the family's head, and they jump over it. They are successful if all members make the jump without getting caught in the rope.
4. If the family is having difficulty making a successful jump, encourage them to discuss and attempt new strategies such as changing their positions or line-up, giving the turners specific directions on how they want the rope turned.

Variations to Family Jump Rope

- ☐ The family sets a goal on how many successive jumps they can make as the rope is continued to be circled around them.
- ☐ The family jumps into the middle, one-by-one, as the rope is being turned.
- ☐ The family jumps into the middle of the circling rope by pairs, trios, or all at the same time.

Family We-Play*

Family We-Play is recommended for all family groups. The only caution for use would be for individuals who have a strong disliking for expressing themselves through physical gestures.

Goals

☐ To break the ice and have some fun.
☐ To identify those things that the family enjoys doing together.

Materials Required

None

Procedures

1. The group stands in a circle facing one another. Each family member thinks of something that she or he enjoys doing with her or his family. It could be a hobby, sport, or another recreational activity. It should be something that can be presented nonverbally as a mime or charade.
2. Demonstrate Family We-Play by jumping into the center of the circle, announcing your name, and acting out your favorite family activity. The rest of the group attempts to guess what you are acting out, similar to what is done in the game of Charades.
3. Following the group's guess and solution, all the other group members, at the same time, jump into the middle of the circle and repeat or mimic, as closely as possible, your name and favorite family activity.
4. The participants then get the opportunity to try this activity. Each participant can take a turn jumping into the middle of the circle, announcing his or her name, and acting out his favorite family activity. The others should follow each person with similar actions.

*Suggested in Fuegelman's (1981) More New Games as "Instant Replay".

Make Beliefs: A Gift For & From Your Family

Make Beliefs encourages family members to view their family world differently, to see possibilities and make new choices. It is based on the assumption that each family member has the power to realize that there is more than one way to view their family, that there are many opportunities for family healing (Zimmerman, 1992). Make Beliefs is a fairly nonthreatening assessment tool that can be used with any number of family participants or families at any point during the program.

Goals

☐ To tap into and examine family's strengths, hopes, and dreams.

Materials Required

Make Beliefs Workbook

Procedure

1. Give each participant a workbook with the following page headings, one assignment per page:

   ☐ Make believe you could create your own set of family holidays. What would they celebrate?

   ☐ Make believe you could reinvent your family life. How would you picture your past?

   ☐ Make believe you created your own sweet blessing for someone in your family. What would it be?

   ☐ Make believe you left a nice message for someone you love deeply. What would it say?

   ☐ Make believe you could dream any dream for your family. What would you dream?

   ☐ Make believe you could catch a favorite moment in your family's life. Which would it be?

   ☐ Make believe that you could snap your fingers and you could change your family. What would they become?

   ☐ Make believe you could wave a magic wand for your family. What two wishes would come true for your family?

   ☐ Make believe you had a golden treasure box. What family treasures would you place inside of it?

2. Offer a variety of writing and drawing materials (crayons, pencils, pens, markers, oil pastels, etc.) to the family members. Encourage them to find their own

spot and take some time to write or draw their responses to the Make Beliefs. If there are individuals in the group who cannot read, someone else can read the Make Beliefs, and the individual can draw in or dictate his or her responses. After completion of the workbook, facilitate the sharing of the family members' responses.

Family-Building Initiatives

Purpose

Family-building initiatives are the core of the experiential program. They are contrived group games that provide participants with concrete experiences, and require communication, problem-solving, cooperation, and personal involvement. The purpose of the initiatives is to create an environment in which the family member's needs and concerns can surface. The family-building initiatives can and should be used as metaphors for the family's daily living situations. They should raise issues for discussion and create a forum where these issues can be resolved.

Strategies for Selecting Family Building Initiatives

Family building initiatives should be strategically selected so that they have the potential to address the family's strengths, concerns, and problems metaphorically. The following page describes some specific guidelines for selecting the initiative exercises.

Guidelines for Selecting Family-Building Initiatives

When selecting games or initiatives for a family session, the counselor should attempt to select those games or initiatives that have the potential to achieve positive responses to the following questions.

_____ Will the game or initiative match the mental, physical, emotional, and maturity levels of the participating family members?

_____ Will the games or initiatives be culturally appropriate for the family participants?

_____ Will the family members stay physically and psychologically safe?

_____ Will the game or initiative be inclusive? Does it have something to offer each family member?

_____ Will the game or initiative encourage family members to take positive, growth-promoting actions?

_____ Will the game or initiative promote creativity, flexibility, spontaneity, and fun?

_____ Will the game or initiative encourage the family participants to use their strengths and resources?

_____ Will the game or initiative assist the family members in gaining new insights about their behaviors, thoughts, attitudes, and feelings?

_____ Will the family members get the opportunity to work on their own goals?

_____ Will the game or initiative produce feelings of having accomplished something?

Strategies for Using the Family-Building Initiatives

The following strategies can assist the practitioner in using the family-building initiatives in a manner that best promotes the well-being and growth of the participants.

Emphasize Physical and Psychological Safety

The physical and psychological safety of the family participants are the primary concern. An exercise should be stopped if the participants become physically exhausted or too emotional, stressed, or tense during the exercise.

Initially Use Initiatives to Break Down Barriers

During the introductory counseling sessions, the families are presented with a series of not-so-threatening initiative activities. These activities are designed to assist the participants in becoming more comfortable with the program and one another, to relieve their initial anxieties, to establish an atmosphere of support, and to build trust in self and the other family participants.

Focus on the Process

The process, not the product, is the key to successful counseling sessions. It is not so important that a family finishes an exercise as it is that they learn from the processes that occur during it. The facilitator should stress this with the family participants.

Use Time-Outs

The exercises have been designed to elicit information about and to change the family's patterns of interactions. Time-outs or pauses should be initiated to discuss and process information that emerges during the exercise. When powerful issues and positive interactions emerge, a time-out should be called to acknowledge and process them.

End An Initiative When It Is Not Working

An exercise should be "stopped" and a new exercise introduced:

- ☐ When an exercise is not working and a family isn't into it.
- ☐ When an exercise becomes much too difficult and begins to cause excess frustration.

Focus on Fun and Enjoyment

Families with problems typically don't have fun together. During the counseling sessions, fun and enjoyable activities are intermixed with the more serious therapeutic interventions. The emphasis on fun and enjoyment helps the family increase their enjoyment in being with one another and the probability that the family will engage in fun activities outside of the counseling setting.

Identify Family Strengths

The feedback given to the families is also directed towards the positive aspects of the family. The family and family observers (other families and counselors) are encouraged to identify the strengths of the family unit and individual family members. Strengths are identified in the areas of communication patterns, interactional styles, and problem-solving techniques. O'Hanlon (1994) recommends, "Find the client's areas of competence, interest, and pleasure, get the details of these, and highlight and expand them" (p. 66).

Use the Family-Building Initiatives as Metaphors

The family-building initiatives should be used as metaphors for the family's daily living situations and to raise relevant issues for discussion (Stitch & Senior, 1984). Carefully designed family-building initiatives fit the unique characteristics, styles, problems, strengths, and positions of the family. Metaphoric transfer occurs when the counseling processes matches or is parallel to the family's real life experiences. "Appropriate framing enhances the therapeutic value of the adventure experience, enabling it to be more prescriptive and specific in application and use" (Gillis, & Gass, 1993, p. 281).

The initiatives are designed to change both the presenting problem and the underlying interactional sequences that maintain it. Once the problem is defined and the interactional sequence that maintains the problem is identified, the counselor formulates a treatment strategy, consisting of an overall plan to use the initiatives as tactical interventions. The repetition of unhealthy and unproductive sequences and interactions is prevented through the introduction of alternatives within the context of the family initiatives (Haley, 1976).

Emphasize Solutions, Not Problems

> It is easier and more profitable to construct solutions than to dissolve problems. It is also easier to repeat already successful behavior patterns than it is to try to stop or change existing problematic behavior. Furthermore, [. . .] activities that center around [sic] finding solutions are distinctively different from problem-solving activities (Berg, 1994, p. 10).

During the experiential exercises, the observable behaviors of the family are emphasized. Explanations of inferential, linear causations are avoided (Heath & Ayers, 1988). Processing or debriefing sessions revolve around discussing what worked for the family rather than what isn't working for them (Davis, 1987). The family focuses on what can be done in the present that is working for them to create a more satisfying family environment.

Identify and Disrupt Problematic Patterns

Often the methods that the family uses in their attempts to solve problems maintain or perpetuate the problem behaviors (Heath & Ayers, 1988). Because the experiential activities present the family members with a variety of problems, their typical problem-solving methods can be directly observed and identified. The patterns of actions and events that make up and surround their difficulties are enacted during the exercises (O'Hanlon, 1994). The methods that the family uses to solve problems provide the direction for the therapeutic planning and intervention (Heath & Ayers, 1988). During the execution of the experiential activities, the family's repetitive and nonworking behavioral and communication patterns are identified and interrupted (O'Hanlon, 1994; Stanton & Todd, 1982). The family analyzes their nonworking attempts to solve problems (Heath & Ayers, 1988).

As the family participates in the initiatives, the counselor and the family members observe the actions and contextual cues that keep the nonworking patterns going. They identify several points where interventions can occur to break the non-working patterns. With the assistance of the larger group of counselors and other families, the family discusses and develops new methods for communication and new alternatives to solve problems. They then get the opportunity to practice these new, healthier alternatives within the context of additional experiential exercises, and later, explore their effectiveness. The cycle is repeated, try an action-based alternative within the context of an initiative, analyze its effectiveness, and try another, possibly healthier action or repeat one that has worked.

Process the Family-Building Initiatives

After completion of the family-building initiatives, the counselor leads the family group in a processing session. Individuals' experiences with the initiatives are almost like fingerprints. Each person develops her or his own patterns of thoughts, feelings, perceptions, and opinions about the experiences. Processing encourages the participants to reflect upon, analyze, describe, and discuss their experiences. They become conscious and better understood. Learning is not left up to chance. Discoveries made during the processing sessions often act as the catalyst for change in the future. Processing increases the opportunities for transfer to real life settings.

> Learning occurs through active extension and grounding of ideas and experiences in the external world, and through internal reflection about the attributes of the experiences and ideas. Processing enhances the richness of the experience, so it stands out and apart, like the important lines of a page underlined with a yellow highlighter (Luckner & Nadler, 1997, p. 10).

Processing assists participants in generalizing the counseling experiences to other settings. When the counseling experience is processed, dissected, analyzed, integrated, and internalized, participants begin to realize they have more choices and influence in their lives (Luckner & Nadler, 1997).

Family-building initiatives can be found on the following pages. Each Family-Building Initiative described in this book has suggestions for processing that initiative.

The Family Juggle

This is a good introductory initiative. It is fun and challenging, and it assists the family participants in getting oriented to the experiential exercises. It can be used with single families or with multifamily groups. The minimum number of participants is five.

Goals

☐ To have the family work on a cooperative venture.
☐ To have the family discover that doing things the same way, in the same pattern, can be counterproductive.

Materials Required

☐ Four or five balls (e.g., koosh balls, tennis balls, etc.)
☐ Stop-watch

Procedures

1. Ask the family group to form a circle. Give one family member a ball and ask her to toss the ball to another member on the other side of the circle. The ball is then tossed to another member and then another until all members have received the ball only one time. Instruct them to remember from whom they received the ball and to whom they passed it. In other words, they create a pattern or sequence of passing and receiving with each member receiving the ball only once. For example, if the ball went from father to daughter to mother to youngest son to oldest son, then the balls must always go in that order and end with father. The family group is asked to practice this sequence several times, always keeping the same pattern of people.

2. Add two or three more balls, one at a time, with the goal being the same to keep the same pattern and have all balls end with the person who began the Family Juggle.

3. After a few practice sessions, tell the family that they will be timed and that the object is to complete the initiative in the least amount of time possible. To do this, give the following two guidelines:

   (a) you should not drop the balls. If you do, a 3-second penalty per dropped ball will be added onto their final time, and

   (b) the balls must always go to the group members in the same order/pattern (the word "throw" should be avoided).

4. Ask the family to designate a person to yell "Go" at the start of their Family Juggle and "Stop" when the starter has gotten all the balls back. Time each attempt for the family. After each attempt, encourage and cajole the family group to reduce their time.

5. Either by trial and error or by careful questioning (e.g., "What can you change to decrease your time?" or "What can you do differently that will reduce your time?"), the family discovers that they can physically change their position in the circle and stand side-by-side in the same order/pattern they originally set up and hand the balls from member to member to reduce their time.

Processing the Family Juggle

Processing of this family initiative revolves around the topic of breaking rigid patterns of doing and thinking. Processing can be directed towards having the family discuss how problems are maintained by always doing things the same way they have always been done (similar to always standing in the same place in the circle). It is based on the concept, "If you always do what you've always done, you always get what you've always gotten and change can occur if you do something differently, anything differently when confronted with a recurring problem."

Cautions

Younger members may get a little excited and throw the balls too hard at the other participants. This would be a good time to stop the group and discuss safety.

The Nurturing Spoons

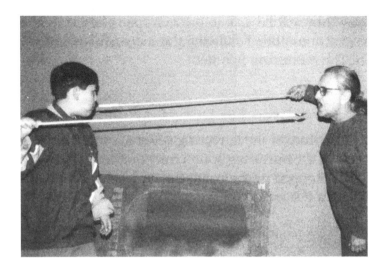

This exercise is suitable for families and groups of families with upper elementary-school-age children and older. It is a nonthreatening initiative that allows families, through a fun activity, to examine the power of a group. It can be used with single families or with multifamily groups. There is no minimum or maximum number of participants needed.

Goal

To have family members realize the importance of nurturing other family members and being nurtured by them.

Materials Required

- ☐ A "nurturing spoon" for each participant (a "nurturing spoon" is a 3-foot long, 1/4" dowel with a spoon [hard plastic or metal] taped onto one end and a piece of colored tape or duct tape taped on the other end).
- ☐ A food substance such as M & M's or Skittles.

Procedures

1. If working with more than one family, ask each family to form their own group or circle. Give each family member a "nurturing spoon." Place a bowl of M & M's or Skittles central to the family group (each family should get a bowl if working with a multigroup format).
2. Simply announce to the family, "Your goal is to eat two spoonfuls of food using the nurturing spoon. You can only use one hand to hold the nurturing spoon and that hand must remain on the taped end opposite the spoon. You will have completed this task when all family members have eaten two spoonfuls of food."

3. After a few moments of struggling, participants realize that since the nurturing spoon is longer than their arms, they will not be able to reach their own mouths. The only way they will be able to eat two spoonfuls of food and complete the task is to feed one another. Following the successful completion of this task, tell the Story of The Nurturing Spoons.

Cautions

Because of the toy-like nature of the nurturing spoons, some kids may try to force-feed their siblings . . . shoving the nurturing spoon into another person's mouth. This action should be immediately stopped by the counselor. A teaching moment is created as the counselor can facilitate a discussion on the importance of creating safety for true nurturing to occur.

Processing The Nurturing Spoons

Processing The Nurturing Spoons involves reading *The Story of the Nurturing Spoons* and asking the participants to discuss the activity and the story.

The Story of The Nurturing Spoons

A person was struggling to understand the difference between heaven and hell. He asked for a guide to help him. A guide appeared and said, "I will help you. I will take you on two journeys." On their first journey they arrived at a place where a great number of family members were seated around a large table. They were all very emaciated and looked near death because of starvation. There was a large bowl of porridge in the center of the table. They were trying to eat, but could not feed themselves because the spoons were longer than their arms, and they could not put the food into their mouths. The guide said, "This is hell."

For their second journey, they arrived at a place where again a great number of family members were seated around a large table. They looked well-fed and happy. There was a large bowl of porridge in the middle of the table. These people were using the same spoons, the ones too long to reach into their own mouths. The difference was they were feeding one another. The guide turned to the person and said, "This is heaven."

Family Pick-Up Sticks

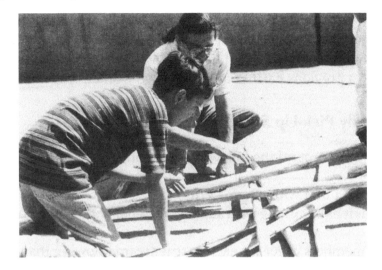

This exercise can be used with families with children of any age. It is best used after a few introductory activities because of the teamwork required and because it asks families to explore their existing subsystems. It can be used with single families or with multifamily groups. There is no minimum or maximum number of participants needed.

Goals

- ☐ To assist the family in working as a cooperative unit.
- ☐ To have the family members explore how family subsystems can benefit the family-as-a-whole.

Materials Required

About a dozen or more 12' to 15' sticks or poles (roughly 3" diameter)

Set-Up

The dozen or so poles are placed in a random stack or pile in a manner similar to the small bundle of sticks that is created when playing the children's game of Pick-Up Sticks.

Procedures

1. Instruct the family: "Your task is to pick up all the sticks or poles. It is similar to the child's game of Pick-Up Sticks, but with big sticks. To do so, you must pick up each pole one at a time, and no other poles can move when you do so."
2. Continue instructions: "Because of the size of the poles, you are being asked to work in partner teams. The other members will act as spotters and tell you if

any of the other poles move. If you are told that another pole has moved, you must immediately drop the pole you were trying to remove. You also must pick a different partner for each round. For example, if dad and oldest son, mom and daughter, and two youngest sons are partners during the first round, they must choose someone different to work with during the second round. You can go back to a previous partner after you have worked with someone else."

Processing Family Pick-Up Sticks

Processing can revolve around the following questions:

- ☐ Who worked best with whom? Why?
- ☐ What was it like working with a family member with whom you typically don't "work?"
- ☐ Did the members cheer for each partner team knowing that it would benefit the whole family team or was each partner team out for themselves?
- ☐ What subsystems exist in the family? Do they benefit or hinder the health of the family?

Cautions

Since this exercise assists the family in exploring their subsystem alliances, caution needs to be used if the subsystem alliances are too strong, or if it is too threatening for a family to explore them at this point in their counseling treatment. For example, families of incest (e.g., father-abused daughter) may not be ready to explore the father/daughter alliance or lack thereof.

Family Parts

This exercise is suitable for families with children of any age. It is best used after a few introductory activities because of the teamwork required and because it asks families to explore the parts members play in their family. It can be used with single families or with multifamily groups. Family units need to have at least three or four people for this activity.

Goals

- ☐ To assist the family in working as a cooperative unit.
- ☐ To have the family members explore what parts or roles they play in the family.

Materials Required

- ☐ Balloons
- ☐ A 20' "soft" field (e.g., a grassy area)

Procedure

1. Give the family a deflated balloon and the following instructions: "As a family unit, you are being asked to blow up a balloon, tie it, cross over this 20-foot area, and break the balloon on the other side. Each of you will be allowed to play only one body part. You will have to decide who will play what parts. In other words, one of you will be one leg, another will be the other leg, another will be an arm and hand and yet another will be the other arm and hand, and one of you will have to be the mouth. After you decide who will play what parts, only the person specified as the mouth will be allowed to speak. You, as a family, can only use your decided upon body parts to blow up the balloon, cross the area, and burst the balloon. Because all family members are challenged in some manner, you can accomplish these tasks only if you become a single unit remaining in direct and constant physical contact."
2. If there are less than five family members, members can play more than one part, but those parts must be different parts of the body (e.g., one leg and a mouth, a mouth and an arm).
3. If there are more than five family members or several families are combined, they can be allowed to have additional legs, arms and mouths. Typically, more people necessitate that more legs are designated to cross over the 20' area.

Cautions

The counselor should ensure that the group is ready for both the teamwork and physical components of this initiative, such as touching, physical moving across an area on one foot, etc.

Processing Family Parts

Processing questions are based on the parts played by the family members during the initiative. Family members can be asked if they typically play that part in their family. For example, if the father was one leg, he can be asked if he is usually the family's quiet strength. If one of the kids was allowed to be the mouth, the family can be asked if he or she is usually the mouth in the family. Usually there is a lot of laughing as members explore how the parts they played in the initiative match the parts they play in their family.

Family Knots*

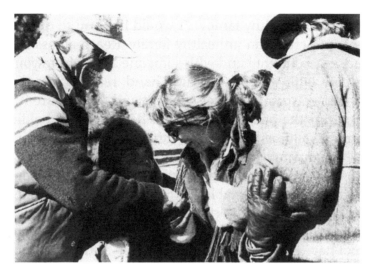

This activity is best used after a few warm-up activities. It is fun and challenging, and it assists the family participants in understanding the initiatives as metaphors for their family experiences. It can be used with single families or with multifamily groups, although the minimum number of participants is eight.

Goals

- ☐ To identify the characteristics of a healthy family.
- ☐ To identify the characteristics of an unhealthy family.
- ☐ To use the characteristics of a healthy family in a problem-solving situation.

Materials Required

None

Procedures

1. Form groups of 8–12 individuals. If working with a large group, several smaller groups of 8–12 can be formed. Family units should be kept intact within the smaller groups. The group is asked to face one another in a hand-holding-hand circle.
2. Introduce the task: "This hand-holding-hand circle represents a healthy family. Based on what you are seeing and feeling, describe the characteristics of a healthy family." Then elicit responses from the participants. If they are having difficulty coming up with characteristics, the counselor can ask additional questions such as: "How do healthy families communicate with one another?" "How do healthy

*Suggested by: Betsy Webb & Christian Itin

families resolve conflicts?" "How do healthy families express affection?" "What are personal boundaries like in healthy families?"

3. Then set up an unhealthy family: "I would like you to drop your hands. Now, we are going to create an unhealthy family. Reach across the circle with your right hand, grasp a right hand with someone across from you, and don't let go. Then, without letting go of your right hand, reach across the circle with your left hand and grasp someone else's left hand. Make sure it is not the person next to you nor the person who's right hand you are holding. At this point, each person should be holding two different hands. As you can see you have formed a human tangle, a symbol of an unhealthy family."

4. Ask the group about the characteristics of an unhealthy family. "I know that many of you are uncomfortable in this hand-in-hand tangle, but being in an unhealthy family is not comfortable. As you think about how you are feeling at the moment, describe the characteristics of an unhealthy family." Groups typically do not have trouble with this description as they describe their feelings of being pressured, having no space or boundaries, and not being able to see one another clearly.

5. Introduce the next phase of the initiative, "Now your goal is to become a healthy family again. In other words, you must unwind your tangle and get back into the healthy family configuration (a hand-in-hand circle) without letting go of hands. You can best do this by using those characteristics you described for a healthy family. Hands may pivot on one another, but contact should not be lost."

6. Let the family struggle with this for awhile and then engage in some stop-action interventions. A sample counselor statement is: "I would like you to become a 'freeze frame' for a moment. Stop what you are doing without letting go. Now, tell me what you have been doing that is characteristic of a healthy family." After a few responses, the group is told that they may continue with their task. The counselor repeats this intervention several times during this initiative.

7. If the group is really struggling with becoming untangled, mention that families sometimes get into such a tangled knot that they need outside assistance, but it is the responsibility of the family to ask for help. If the group asks for help, the counselor tells the group that they can separate one pair of hands within the group and regrasp them anywhere they like. The group should be encouraged to decide by consensus which pair of hands should be selected.

8. Because of the initial grasping configuration, two or three circles may form or some people may face out while others face into the circle. This is okay, and the group should still view these situations as successes.

Cautions

The major risk of Family Knots is that it asks the participants to make close physical contact. Thus, major care should be used in families where physical violence or sexual abuse has been or is an issue.

Processing Family Knots

Most of the processing occurs throughout the initiative as the counselor questions the group about the characteristics of healthy and unhealthy families. After the initiative, the group can further discuss and analyze these characteristics as well as make some comparisons to their own families.

The Family Jewels

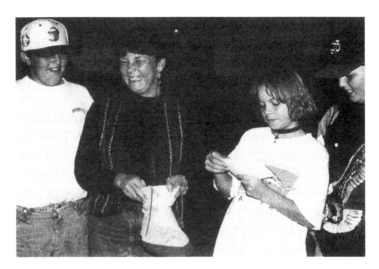

This is best used after a few warm-up activities. It is fun and challenging, and it assists the family participants in understanding the use of the initiatives as metaphors for life experiences. It is designed to be used with multifamily groups.

Goals

- ☐ To identify those qualities about their family that they would not want to lose.
- ☐ To learn that some tasks cannot be done alone, and that assistance from other family members may be needed.
- ☐ To learn to ask for help from other family members.

Materials Required

- ☐ Index cards
- ☐ Writing utensils
- ☐ A large sock or stocking (a leftover Christmas stocking works well)

Procedures

1. This initiative may be introduced as follows: "This exercise is called The Family Jewels. First, I would like your family to identify your family's jewels by writing on the index cards those special qualities about your family that you would not like to lose, one special quality per index card." Each family group makes its own stack of family index cards which identifies their strengths.
2. After the family finishes this task, ask them to share these qualities with the counselor and the other families. The counselor places one "volunteer" family's cards into the stocking and places the stocking on the ground.
3. Introduce the next phase: "I have placed those special family qualities into the

stocking for extra protection. If you are like most families, you would probably do most anything to protect these special qualities from adverse forces, from forces that can take away your Family Jewels (so-to-speak). Usually, there is one member of the family that puts more effort and energy into protecting the Family Jewels than the other members. Please take a minute and identify who that person is." (Note: I keep these directions vague and allow the family to define the meaning of "effort and energy.")

4. After a family decides who is the Protector of the Family Jewels, continue: "This family member is the Protector of the Family Jewels. Now, I would like you, as a large group, to identify all those Adverse Forces that can steal the Family Jewels." As Adverse Forces such as unemployment, drug and alcohol addiction, and mental health difficulties are identified, the members from the other families are asked to play these roles. For example, dad from another family may volunteer to play alcoholism. (Note: If the number of players are at a minimum, members of the Protector's family can play some of the Adverse Forces. If there is an adequate number of members from other families, about 6–8 people, then the Protector's family should observe the next phase of the exercise.)

5. The counselor continues: "The members from the other families will act as the Aversive Forces and attempt to take away the Family Jewels. The job of the Protector of the Family Jewels is to prevent the jewels from being snatched away by the Adverse Forces. The only way that the Adverse Forces can be stopped is for the Protector of the Family Jewels to tag them before they can grab the Family Jewels. The Jewel Protector can stand near the Family Jewels, but cannot stand on them or hold onto them. If an Adverse Force is tagged, he or she must move away from the playing area. The game ends when all the Adverse Forces are tagged and frozen or when one of them has taken the Family Jewels."

6. More than likely, the Family Jewels/stocking will be snatched away before all the Adverse Forces are tagged because the other members will outnumber the one Family Jewels Protector. If this happens, it is interesting to note which Adverse Force snatched away the Family Jewels.

7. This scenario also sets the scene for the next phase of the activity: "It appears that the task of protecting the Family Jewels by oneself is quite difficult. Protecting the Family Jewels is often a family affair. Protector of the Family Jewels, would you like some assistance with your task? If so, ask any or all of your family members to help you by becoming additional Protectors."

8. The game is played the same way as before, but now with additional Protectors of the Family Jewels. With the added members, it becomes difficult, if not impossible for the Adverse Forces to snatch away the Family Jewels.

9. The other families should get a chance to protect their Family Jewels, beginning the process again with one Protector of the Family Jewels, asking for help, if needed, etc.

Cautions

The major risk of The Family Jewels exercise is that it asks the participants to become active in a running activity. Participants may become physically aggressive while trying to protect or snatch away the Family Jewels. If this is the case, the counselor should stop the activity and discuss safety issues.

Processing The Family Jewels

Depending on the family's goals and the behaviors observed during the exercise, processing topics can include:

- ☐ Identifying adverse forces in the family's life.
- ☐ Identifying methods to overcome the adverse forces and protect the family's special qualities.
- ☐ Examining what it was like asking for help from other family members.
- ☐ Identifying situations when family members should ask for help from one another.

Family Tower of Power

This exercise is suitable for families with children of elementary school age and older. It is a nonthreatening activity that allows families to recognize, articulate, and build on their strengths.

Goal

To have the family identify their strengths and create a metaphoric tower that represents those strengths.

Materials Required

- ☐ Index cards of various sizes
- ☐ Popsicle sticks
- ☐ Tape, glue
- ☐ Markers

Procedures

1. Provide each family group with index cards of various sizes, popsicle sticks, markers, and glue or tape and introduce the task: "You will now get the opportunity to build a Family Tower of Power. You will be judged on creativity and structural soundness. You can use any of the available index cards and popsicle sticks, but you must first earn them by writing a family strength on each item. I will throw in the tape and glue for free. You will also be asked to explain how each member made a contribution to the building of the Family Tower of Power."
2. After completion of the towers, give the family the opportunity to describe their tower as well as the contributions of each member. If working in a multigroup setting, the entire group can go on a neighborhood tour, so that each family gets a chance to describe their tower to the others.

Cautions

The risks with this activity are very low, but families in extreme chaos or distress may be unwilling or unable to identify their strengths.

Processing The Family Tower

Processing occurs as each family gets the opportunity to describe their tower and their strengths.

Chain Reaction

(Conceptualized by Gina Griego)

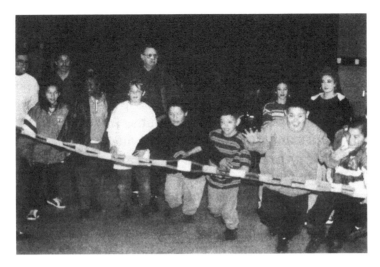

This exercise is suitable for families with children of any age. It works especially well with elementary school children because of its arts and crafts component. It is best used after a few introductory activities because it asks the family to identify possible problem behaviors in the family. It can be used with single families or with multifamily groups. There is no minimum or maximum number of participants needed.

Goal

- ☐ To assist families in exploring how the behavior of one family member can affect other family members.
- ☐ To have the family members identify ways to break the chain of negative behavioral patterns.

Materials Required

- ☐ Materials to make paper chains (construction paper, scissors, paste or tape)
- ☐ Markers

Procedures

1. Introduce the task: "You are going to make a paper chain out of construction paper similar to the paper chains kids make in school. So to begin, please cut the construction paper into strips that are eleven inches long and three inches wide."
2. After the strips are cut, give the following directions: "This chain is going to be a little different than the ones kids make in school. Label the first link of the chain with an unhealthy or problematic behavior of one family member. Some

examples may include: (a) getting in trouble at school or at work, (b) getting in trouble with the law, (c) drug or alcohol use, (d) getting into fights, (e) stealing, or (f) being aggressive with other family members."

3. "After the behavior is written on a strip of construction paper, join the two ends to form the first link. Next, identify at least one negative consequence on each family member as a result of that behavior. For example, mom may state that her daughter's troubles at school cause her to lose sleep at night, or son may state that dad's drinking causes him not to be able to concentrate at school. Write these consequences on the paper strips, create links and join them to the first link so that a long paper chain results. Try to see how long you can make the chain by identifying any and all consequences of that one behavior."

4. After the chain is formed and the information on the chain is discussed and processed by the family, give the following directions: "We have seen how one member's behavior can create a chain reaction. But you, as a family, also have the power to break the chain. We (two people not in the family) will hold up the chain by its two ends. Each one of you is to state one way you can break this chain of negative consequences. Once all of you have identified how you will break the chain, you, as a group, will gather on one side of the chain, count to three, and then run through the paper chain, tearing it to bits."

Caution

When the participants identify problematic behaviors in their family, emotional distress may result. The counselor should be ready to intervene and process the exercise if members are becoming too upset.

Processing Chain Reaction

The processing should focus on what it felt like to break the chain, and how the family members plan to break similar chains in the future.

▨ The Family Strengths Protector

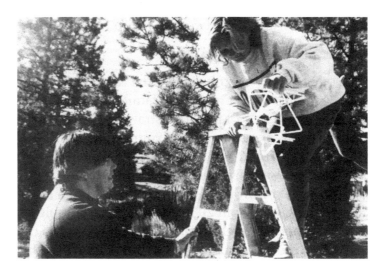

This activity is best used after a few introductory activities because it requires family teamwork and cooperation. Although this initiative can be used with single families or with multifamily groups, it works most effectively in a setting that uses a multifamily group format.

Goals

- ☐ To highlight the family's strengths.
- ☐ To identify and develop some means to protect the family's strengths.
- ☐ To examine the effects of stress on the family system.

Materials Required

- ☐ Each family group needs crayons, a raw egg, 25 plastic straws, and about 35" of masking tape.
- ☐ An 8' or taller step ladder (if indoors, a drop cloth to catch eggs).

Procedures

1. Identifying Family Strengths

   a. Distribute the eggs and crayons to each family and give the following introduction: "This initiative is called The Family Strengths Protector. Discuss all those family strengths and characteristics that you would not want to lose, those things that make your family special. Make sure that each family member has an opportunity to state his or her opinion. Write these strengths on the egg with the crayons."

   b. Bring out the straws and set up the next phase by saying: "Now, discuss all of the behaviors, skills, and coping mechanisms that your family members can use to protect the family's strengths. The straws represent these protective mechanisms. Every time that you tell me one of your family's protective mechanism, you will receive two straws (up to 25 straws)."

2. Creating the Family Strengths Protector

   a. After the distribution of straws, give the families 35" of masking tape and tell them: "Your task is to create, as a family unit, a Family Strengths Protector using the straws and tape. The straws and masking tape are the only materials that you can use to protect your family strengths-egg. The purpose of the Strengths Protector Mechanism is to prevent the cracking of the family's strengths—the egg—when it is subjected to stress and sudden shock. The egg and its carrier will be dropped onto the floor from a ladder."

   b. The families are given about 20 to 30 minutes to complete their designs. The counselor ensures that each family has enough time to create their egg protector unit and then asks all families to gather around the ladder.

3. Subjecting the Family Strengths Protector to External Stressors

   a. Describe the next phase: "The ladder represents external stressors in a family's life. These are the stressors that can weaken or crack your family's strengths. Your family will present your Family Strengths Protector to the rest of the group by: (1) describing your family's strengths, and (2) deciding, as a family, how far up the ladder you will go to drop your Family Strengths Protector/Egg. The higher up you go on the ladder, the more stress you will place on the family's strengths/egg and the greater chance that it will crack. You will be allowed to drop the egg as many times as you choose as long as the egg stays intact. In other words, you have the option to begin testing the effects of stress on your family's strengths by dropping it while standing on the lower ladder rungs and then working your way up to the higher rungs. This method will allow you to examine how small increments of stress affect your family strengths."

   b. Give each family an opportunity to present their Family Strengths Protector. The counselor "spots" (as in gymnastics) the family member who drops the egg from the ladder.

Cautions

Minimal risks exist for this exercise, but families in extreme chaos or distress may be unwilling or unable to identify their strengths.

Processing The Family Strengths Protector

Most of the processing occurs as the families discuss their strengths, their protective mechanisms, and the effects of stress on their family. Some questions that can be used during the activity include:

☐ Who (which family member) stated which strengths?
☐ What do you, as other families, think are the strengths of this family?
☐ What are some of the skills you, as a family, believe will protect your strengths?
☐ What are some additional skills and behaviors that you will need to use in the future to protect your family's strengths?
☐ What types of stress are common for your family? What types of stress are anticipated in the future?

After the activity, the counselor can focus on some of the following issues

☐ Those times when the tape and straws are most needed, times in the family's life when high stress levels demand the use of effective coping mechanisms to protect its strengths.
☐ How each individual family member can best use the tape and straws (i.e., the family's positive coping mechanisms).
☐ What the family can do if their strengths become weakened and cracked.

The Family Obstacle Field

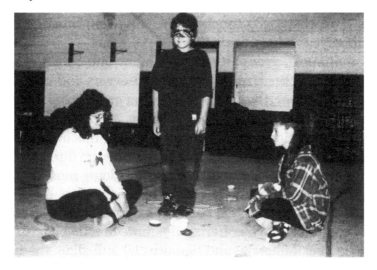

This initiative is most appropriate following a few introductory initiatives because it requires a fair amount of communication and trust. It can be used with single families or multifamily groups.

Goals

- ☐ To establish a hierarchy in which parents are in charge.
- ☐ To create an opportunity for the child to listen to directions provided by his or her parents.
- ☐ To have the parents (if both are participating) work as a team in giving directions to their child(ren).

Materials Required

- ☐ Lots of obstacles—tennis balls, ping pong balls, rubber chickens, frisbees, etc.
- ☐ Blindfolds

Procedures

1. Establish a boundary area of 40 feet by 10 feet. Scatter the obstacles throughout the field. Younger children may be asked to help spread out the obstacles. Direct the parent(s) to stand at one end of the field and the children at the other end (See variations for alternatives).
2. Introduce the task: "A major responsibility of parenting is to guide children through the obstacles of life with as few bumps and bruises as possible. Children must learn to trust that their parents can lead them through these obstacles even when the children cannot clearly see the way. This initiative is based on these ideas. It is called The Family Obstacle Field. The object is for the parent(s) to provide verbal directions to guide their blindfolded child(ren)

through the simulated field of life's obstacles. The parents must navigate the child(ren) through the obstacles while remaining at the far end away from the child(ren). If an obstacle is touched, the child(ren) must go back to the start, and the initiative is begun again."

3. If using a multifamily group, it is best to allow one family at a time to attempt the initiative. The other families become observers and obstacles. During and after a family's attempt, the other families can provide feedback to them. (Note: I am always amazed how the other families, even ones with young children, give constant attention to the family attempting this initiative.)

4. Potential Counselor Intervention: If both parents are directing the child through The Family Obstacle Field, one parent may be doing most of the directing while the other remains passive and silent. If this is the case, the counselor can stop the initiative and inquire if this pattern is typical in other settings. If it is, the counselor can intervene by offering the more directive parent the opportunity to take a step back (literally and figuratively) and allow the quieter, less directive parent to direct the blindfolded child.

5. Variations:

☐ Blindfold all the children and ask the parent(s) to lead them through the obstacle field at the same time.

☐ Inquire about emotionally close parent-child subsystems. Create parent/child dyads that pair up the more distant parent and child. This parent then leads the child through the obstacles while the other parent becomes a silent observer.

☐ If younger children are present, have them act as obstacles while their older sibling is being led through the obstacle field. This creates a metaphor for how the younger sibling can be perceived as an obstacle by an older sibling.

☐ Ask a single parent to lead all of his or her children through the field. This creates a metaphor for the difficulty that one parent has guiding all children through life alone.

Cautions

The counselor needs to be alert to those individuals who have a strong fear reaction to being blindfolded.

Processing The Family Obstacle Field

Processing questions can be based on some of the metaphors developed during the initiative and can include the following topics.

☐ Parents taking charge
☐ The importance of both parents providing similar directions
☐ Children listening to parents
☐ Parents' difficulty seeing from the children's perspective
☐ Parents needing to provide concrete, understandable directions

Crossing the Problem Pit

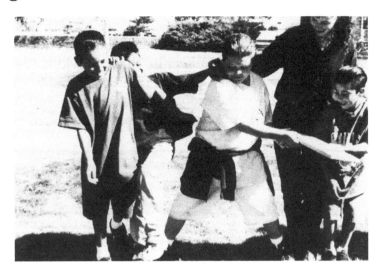

Since this activity asks families to identify their family problems, it is best used after the families have been oriented to the program format, the counselor, and the other families, if a multifamily group. This initiative is designed for use with multifamily groups or for use with single families.

Goals

☐ To identify those problem areas that are having negative effects on the family.
☐ To identify and use those problem-solving skills that will help resolve the problems.

Materials Required

☐ 40 feet of butcher's paper or a 40-foot long sidewalk or parking lot
☐ Magic markers—variety of colors or Chalk—variety of colors (if using sidewalk)
☐ 2- or 3-inch wide masking or mailing tape
☐ 1" × 10" or 2" × 10" boards—lengths ranging from 12" to 20".
(The number of boards is dependent on the number of participants. A good rule of thumb is one board per two to three participants.)

Procedures

1. Identifying the Problem: The Problem Pit area is established either by laying out and anchoring (with tape or heavy objects on the sides) the butcher paper or setting up boundaries of about 3' by 40' on the sidewalk or parking lot. The chalk (for sidewalks) or the magic markers (for paper) should be placed nearby.

   Introduce the task: "This initiative is called Crossing the Problem Pit. First, you will need to identify all those problem areas that cause your family any type of stress or distress. Each family member should have an opportunity to state those problems that he or she believes affect the family. The problems are to be written or drawn out on the butcher block paper or sidewalk, the Problem Pit. Write or draw your problems throughout the entire length of The Problem Pit area using the markers or chalk provided. Each of you should attempt to write or draw at least two or three problems or stressors. After you are done, we walk down the Problem Pit as a group and have all of you describe, if you choose, what you wrote or drew." (See Figure 4.1).

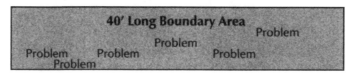

FIGURE 4.1.

If working with a single family, the counselor can accompany the family as they identify their problems. This will give the counselor the opportunity to examine the family dynamics and to provide guiding questions. If using a multifamily group format, all families can work concurrently on identifying and listing their problems. Families should be warned that, after they finish this part of the activity, they will be asked to share, if they choose, their identified problems with the other families. The counselor should spend some time with each family.

Cautions

Some families may have intense emotional reactions to seeing their problems written or drawn out. The counselor should be prepared to provide an intervention if this occurs. The rest of the initiative may have to be put on hold while the family members discuss their feelings and thoughts about their problem areas.

2. Developing Problem-Solving Methods
   This phase involves the use of the boards which are prepared ahead of time. Place a piece of tape lengthwise across the middle of the board. Use indelible magic markers to write out the problem-solving methods on the tape/board set-up.

   Ask the family to identify those general problem-solving methods that can assist them in coping with or alleviating some of their identified problems. Each method is written out on a board with one method per board. (See Figure 4.2.)

   Introduce the next part of the task: "Discuss all those problem-solving methods that you, as a family, can use to help you cope with or alleviate the stress associated with your problems. (Note: I emphasize that not all problems can be totally resolved, e.g., unemployment, but that there are strategies that can be used to reduce the stress associated with them.) You should identify one method at a time. After a method is identified, write it on one of the boards. You have the potential of using ___ number of boards (one board per two to three participants) for the initiative. Thus, if you want to use them all, you will need to identify ___ number of problem-solving methods."

Board #1

FIGURE 4.2.

3. Crossing the Problem Pit
   Explain how the family or families will cross the Problem Pit: "Your task now is to have your family (or families, if a multifamily group) use the problem-solving methods (boards) as stepping stones to cross over the Problem Pit. Your guidelines are:

   a. Only the boards may touch the problem pit. No parts of your body nor any other props can be used.
   b. The problem-solving methods (boards) may be used in a forward movement only towards the end of the Problem Pit. In other words, the boards may not be passed back toward the starting point. (The metaphor is that we want to make forward progress toward problem resolution.)
   c. If a family member touches the ground with any part of his or her body, the entire family group must begin again.

   "To put it simply, you are to use the boards to go from one end of the Problem Pit to the other. You are not permitted to touch the Pit with any body parts or any other props."

   As the family crosses over the Problem Pit, the counselor can ask the family to make connections between the problem-solving methods being used during the initiative and the problem-solving methods the family wrote on the boards. For example, a family may have written on a board that one of their problem-solving methods is "to use each other for support." If the family, while crossing the Problem Pit, is using each other for support while standing on the board that states this method, the counselor can ask the family to make this connection.

   The counselor can take the metaphor one step further by assisting the family in making a connection between using the problem-solving methods and solving their identified problems. The family may have written in the Problem Pit that one of their problems is the "vicious arguing between the two brothers." As the family literally crosses over this statement written in the Problem Pit, the counselor can make a comment such as: "You have crossed over this problem (brothers arguing) by using family support. You have literally crossed over this problem by using one another for support." This will only work, of course, if the brothers have not argued during the initiative. The family can be encouraged to make metaphors such as this one throughout the activity.

Cautions

This activity asks the family to identify their family's problem areas and thus, may be perceived as risky or threatening.

Processing The Problem Pit Crossing

Most of the processing questions occur as the families identify their problems, discuss problem-solving methods, and cross over The Problem Pit. Processing at the end of this initiative is minimal and revolves around what the family learned and what they plan to do differently at home.

Suggested Questions For Use During the Problem Identification Stage

- ☐ What types of problems are your family facing?
- ☐ Each member is asked, "What do you see as this family's greatest problem?"

Suggested Questions For Use During the Development of Problem-Solving Methods

- ☐ When you had a problem as a family in the past, what worked in solving it?
- ☐ What are some problem-solving methods you have used individually but not as a family?
- ☐ What are some problem-solving methods that you think would work, but have not tried?

Suggested Questions For Use During the Crossing the Problem Pit Stage

- ☐ Which methods, written on the boards, are you currently using to cross over the problem pit?
- ☐ Which problem-solving method would work best to solve (the problem that the family is crossing over in the problem pit)?

End of Session Debriefing Questions

- ☐ Which problems do you see yourself being able to solve in the near future? How?
- ☐ How will you use your identified problem-solving methods at home?

Crossing Over Hard Ships

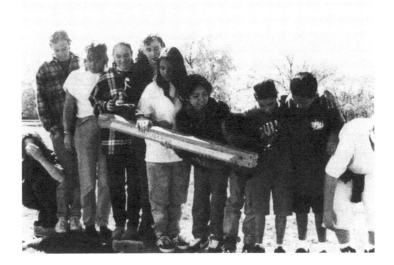

This activity is one of the most difficult in terms of physical demands and the need for problem-solving and teamwork. It is best used after the family has been oriented to the program format, the counselor, and the other families, if applicable. This initiative is appropriate for both multifamily groups and single family sessions.

Goals

- [ ] To describe those past hardships or difficult times that the family has successfully resolved.
- [ ] To describe those hardships or difficult times that the family is currently facing.
- [ ] To identify those resources and supports outside the family that have helped or could help them get over their hardships.
- [ ] To learn how to use external supports and resources most effectively.

Materials Required

- [ ] About a dozen or so cut-out outlines of paper ships
- [ ] 3" wide masking tape
- [ ] Indelible magic markers
- [ ] Four 3" diameter PVC pipes - cut in 36" sections (at hardware store)
- [ ] Three 4" × 4" × 8' boards (sanded down to prevent splinters)
- [ ] One 1" × 36" Hardwood Dowel

Procedures

1. Set-Up
   - [ ] For the Identifying Hard Ships phase, the paper ship cut-outs are needed.
   - [ ] For the Crossing Over Hard Ships phase, a strip of masking tape should be

placed on each of the boards and pipes. These items, along with the dowel, should be placed in a random pile at the beginning point of a 40' long playing field.

2. Identifying Family Hard Ships

The paper ships and markers are needed for this phase of the exercise. Introduce the task: "This exercise is called Crossing Over Hard Ships. First, I would like you to identify those hardships that your family has faced in the past and has successfully resolved. After each hardship is identified, it is to be written on the paper ship. . . one hardship per ship." The family is given time to complete this task. Then, ask the family to identify current hardships: "Now, I would like you to identify those hardships that your family is currently facing. Each one of your current hardships should also be written on the paper ships." If working with multifamily groups, each family should identify their own past and current hardships.

3. Identifying External Resources and Supports

Bring the family to the area where the three boards, four PVC pipes, and the dowel are placed. They are asked to identify the resources and supports that worked in the past to help them get over their hardships: "These items represent the external resources and supports that helped you get over your hardships and difficult times in the past. They can be human, financial, organizational, or any other type of support that helped you get over your hardships. Each time you identify a resource or support, you earn one of these items. After you identify your resource or support, you will label the item with the "name" of that resource or support. It would probably be to your advantage to earn all eight items. As a gift, I'll throw in the dowel for free." If working with multifamily groups, all the families can work together to identify external resources and supports.

4. Setting Up the Hard Ship Field

After the family finishes identifying resources and earning the pipes and boards, set up the Hard Ship Field. Place the "labeled" paper ships in a line in the 40' long playing field in sequential order from past to current hardships: "This is your hard ship field. Place your hard ships in a type of time line across the field with past hardships at the beginning of the field and the current ones closer to the end." (See Figure 4.3.)

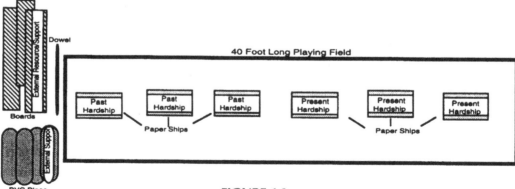

FIGURE 4.3.

5. Crossing Over Hard Ships

Present the family group with the task of getting the entire group across the designated area using only the three boards, the four pipes, and the dowel: "Now, your task is to cross over your hardships by transporting your family group across the designated area using your resources or supports—the available PVC pipes, boards and wooden dowel—without touching the ground with the boards, any body parts, or any other props. Only the pipes and dowel may touch the ground. The general rule is, 'Round can touch the ground, square needs to stay in the air.' If any part of your body or a board touches the ground within the designated area, the entire group will be required to start over. An additional guideline is that no family members can remain at the start while other members are getting off at the end. In other words, all family members must be en route across the designated area before any member can step off at the end. The reason for this guideline is that families often must face and cross over their hardships together rather than alone or in small groups." (See Figure 4.4.)

Solution - Overhead View

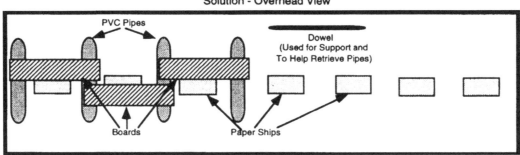

Not Drawn to Scale

FIGURE 4.4.

Safety and Spotting Procedures

☐ This initiative is best done on a soft, grassy playing field so that the pipes don't roll as easily and cause a fall. If done on a hard floor, the pipes should be covered with foam or pipe insulation to offset some of the rolling effects.

☐ Jumping from pipe to pipe is not allowed.

☐ Piggyback riding is not allowed.

☐ Participants should be warned that the pipes may roll when the boards and participants are placed on top. (Note: This warning should occur after the participants develop and begin to implement their solution.)

☐ Participants should be encouraged to give each other a helping hand while crossing over the boards.

Cautions

This activity asks family members to work both physically and emotionally close together, and thus may be perceived as risky or threatening.

Processing Crossing Over the Hardships

Most of the processing occurs: (1) as the family members figure out a method for using the materials to cross over the designated area, and (2) while they are crossing it. As the family struggles to find a working method for using the materials, identify the theme as, "You can have all the resources and supports in the world, but if you don't use them effectively, then they won't work for you." If the family gets stuck, questions should be directed toward assisting the family members in seeing how they can use their resources or supports to solve the problem. For example, ask them "How can you use all of the materials in a systematic and cooperative fashion?" or "How can you bridge the gap between how you *are* using the materials and how you *can* use them?"

As the family crosses over the designated area and thus their hardships, the theme may be around, "How can resources and supports that worked in the past help resolve current hardships?" As the family crosses over past hardships into the area of their present hardships, the counselor can ask how the given resource or support can assist with the resolution of the current hardship. For example, a family may have identified "Johnny's school problems" as a current hardship. They further identified "asking family friends for help" as a resource that helped resolve a past hardship. When the family gets to Johnny's paper hardship, the counselor can ask the family to stop for a moment and discuss how they can use family friends to help with Johnny's school problems.

Following the initiative, the family can: (1) further discuss which external resources and supports can help resolve current difficulties, and (2) develop plans of action that specify how they will use their external resources and supports to resolve their current problems.

The Dumping Field

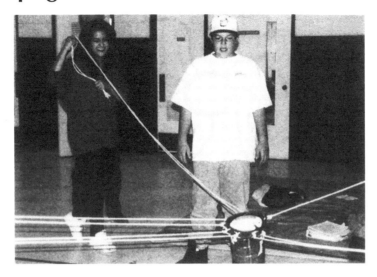

Since this activity requires the family to identify their problems and then work cooperatively as a team, it is best used after the families have been oriented to the program format, the counselor, and the other families, if applicable. This initiative is designed for use with either multifamily groups or for single family sessions.

Goals

☐ To have the family members identify the problem areas that are having negative effects on their family.

☐ To have family members discover that, if they work together, they can dump many of their problems.

Materials Required

☐ #10 cans (the kind that restaurant vegetables come in)—one per family
☐ Trash can
☐ Tape, 1/4" rope or 1/4" PVC pipe to set up boundaries
☐ The Dumping Device (twelve 15' lengths of nylon rope cut and tied into a 6" diameter bicycle inner tube or 1/4" to 1/2" bungee cord)
☐ Index cards of various sizes (3" × 5", 4" × 6", and 5 1/2"× 8")
☐ Assortment of magic markers or crayons

Procedures

1. Set-Up
   A bicycle inner tube (or bungee cord) and nylon cord are needed for the Dumping Device. To make the Dumping Device, cut a 6 1/2" long piece of bicycle tubing or bungee cord. If working with an inner tube, use a hole punch tool to

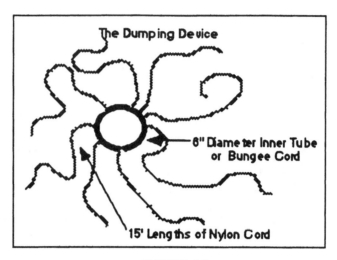

FIGURE 4.5.

punch several holes in both ends of the bicycle tube and tie these ends together with the nylon cord (with a 1/2" overlap so that a 6" diameter rubber circle is created). The alternative to the inner tube set-up is to tie a foot long length of bungee cord together with a water knot or fisherman's knot to form a 6" loop. Then, eight to twelve 15' lengths of nylon cord are cut and tied at equal intervals to the inner tube or bungee cord. (See Figure 4.5.)

Next, set up the dumping field. PVC pipe or 1/4" cord can be used to set up boundaries that measure about 20' by 10'. A trash can is placed inside the boundary near one end, and the Dumping Device is placed on the other end on the outside of these boundaries.

Index cards of various sizes and an assortment of markers are placed in a #10 can. Each family, if a multifamily group, receives this kit.

2. Give the kit containing the index cards, markers, and #10 can to each family to use for the Problem Identification Phase.

3. Problem Identification Phase
Introduce the task: "This initiative is called The Dumping Field. The first part of the initiative requires you to identify any problems currently facing your family. Individually, you are being asked to identify two family problems. Then, your family-as-a-whole should identify two additional problems. The problems are written or drawn out on the index cards, one problem per card. As you can see, in the #10 can there are three different sizes of cards. If you think the problem is a small one, write or draw it on the small index card. If you think it is a very big one, place it on the large card. A medium-size problem goes on the medium size card." After the family members finish writing or drawing out their problems, ask them to read them aloud. They can choose to read aloud any or all of their identified problems. Then, have them put all of the family's cards into their #10 can. (See Figure 4.6.)

4. The Problem Dumping Phase
The next phase involves the use of the Dumping Field. The family's (or a volunteer family's, if working in a multigroup format) #10 can with the problems

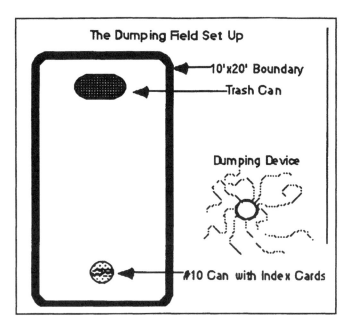

FIGURE 4.6.

inside is placed inside the boundary area on the far end away from the trash can. Introduce this part of the task: "Now you will get the opportunity to dump your problems from the #10 can into the Family Problem Disposal Unit (the trash can). To do so, you will need to use the Dumping Device that you see next to the boundary area. Nothing may enter or leave the boundary except for the Dumping Device. In other words, no body parts nor other props can enter into the boundaries. The #10 can or trash can cannot leave the boundaries. You will have successfully completed this task when you have dumped all of your index cards into the trash can. The #10 can needs to be left outside of the trash can."

As the family struggles to dump the index cards from the #10 can into the trash can, the larger cards often get stuck in the #10 can. This situation provides a scenario to discuss how difficult it is to dump larger problems.

Variations

☐ To add a little spice to the initiative task, family members can be challenged to attempt the task alone (it cannot be done alone), and then later encouraged to ask for help from other family members. This approach is a metaphor for trying to dump family problems alone, rather than seeking the assistance of family members.

☐ If more than one family unit is participating, all the families can place their #10 cans inside of the boundary area. The families can attempt the initiative task one family at a time being careful not to disturb the other families' cans.

☐ A parent-in-charge-of-child challenge can be set up. The children are blind-folded and cannot speak, but can touch the Dumping Device. The parents can see and speak, but cannot touch the Dumping Device nor the children. Parents are paired with children and they must guide the children through the dumping process. This initiative often creates a forum about the need for parents to give children explicit and understandable directions.

Cautions

This activity asks families to identify their family's problem areas and, thus, may be perceived as risky or threatening.

Processing The Dumping Field

Processing can include the following topics:

- ☐ What it takes to dispose of a family's problems.
- ☐ Thoughts and feelings about working as a family unit to dispose of problems.
- ☐ The difference between dumping small problems versus dumping large problems.

T-Shirt Panorama

A Group or Family Initiative

(Conceptualized by Andy Greif)

This exercise is suitable for all ages. It is especially suitable for families who enjoy learning through artistic activities.

Goal:

To have the family create an art response that celebrates the group, or the family unit.

Materials Required

☐   One T-shirt per participant
☐   Several different colors of T-shirt markers or bottles of T-shirt paint

Procedures

1. Lead the family program participants in a discussion about how their family has enriched their personal lives.
2. Lay out T-shirts, equaling the number of participants, in a line to create a long canvas. Give the group the task of drawing or painting onto their T-shirts a panorama that depicts the richness of their family experiences. Their goal is to create an end product that uses all the T-shirts as one canvas.
3. To achieve this, the family or group members line up in front of the shirts, one person per shirt. Each member gets one minute per shirt to add something to the shirt painting with the awareness that the goal is create one big picture out of all of the T-shirts. After a minute passes, the counselor calls "time" and the line moves one shirt to their right with the last person going to the front of the line. This one-minute timing process is continued until each person has had the opportunity to draw on each shirt.
4. All participants are given a T-shirt, a donation from their family group as a reminder of their experiences with the group.

Cautions

None

Processing T-Shirt Panorama

Processing this activity involves acknowledging and celebrating family successes.

Desert Island

This exercise is suitable for all ages. It is especially suitable for families who value and enjoy active, game-like, and concrete ways of learning.

Goal

To provide a concrete example of the benefits of changing patterns of perceiving and doing.

Materials Required

Hoola hoops and bicycle tire inner tubes

Procedures

1. After reading the Desert Island fable (see story after description), introduce the family to the Desert Island Initiative.
2. Lay out several bicycle inner tubes or hoola hoops on the ground to form several loops. The larger the group, the more tubes or hoops that will be needed.
3. Introduce the task: "Your task is to have all of your feet inside the loops. No portion of your feet may touch the loops or extend over, under, or beyond the loops. You will be successful when all of your members have concurrently accomplished this task." (Typical concerns include: "piggy backing" which is not allowed, and having one foot in one loop and the other in another loop, which is allowed as long as each foot is within a loop and not touching it.)
4. After they accomplish this task (which at this point should be fairly easy), take away a loop and give the group the same task. Take away loops away one at a time until there is only one loop left. At this point, the only way the group will be successful is to sit on the ground and place their feet within the tube. One group member almost always discovers this. (Note: The last loop must be a size that will not permit the accomplishment of the task from a standing position.)
5. Most groups will assume that the task must be accomplished in a standing position, but this is never stated in the directions. The family learns that by thinking about things differently and by trying new behaviors, they may achieve helpful new insight and healthier behaviors.

Cautions

This initiative asks family members to be is close physical proximity. The counselor should use caution (or not use the initiative at all) if the family has boundary problems related to physical or sexual abuse.

Processing Desert Islands

The counselor can help the family identify a real life situation or two in which the family feels stuck. They can then brainstorm ways to think and act differently to solve family problems.

The Desert Island

They woke up one morning on a desert island. They had no recollection how they got there. But one thing they knew for certain—the man, woman, and child were stranded. The mainland was visible in the near distance.

The man said, "There is no need to get upset. The mainland is within swimming distance. I'll swim and get help."

He jumped into the water and began to swim only to quickly be pulled back to shore because of the strong tide. Undaunted, he said, "Don't worry. The tide is too strong. We'll try later in the day when it is not so strong."

Later in the day, the tide seemed lower. The woman stated, "I've always been a good swimmer. I'll give it a try." And she jumped into the water and began to swim only to be pulled back to shore because the tide was too strong. She said, "Not to worry. We'll try tomorrow when we are better rested."

Tomorrow came. Both the man and woman tried to swim to the mainland. Both the man and woman were pulled back to shore because the tide was too strong.

Each day, like clockwork, morning, noon, and night, the man and woman would try to swim to the mainland, only to be quickly pulled back to shore because of the strong tide.

The tide also brought many other things into shore as tides tend to do. One day the tide washed in a bottle. The young girl picked up the bottle and found a note in it. The note in the bottle read, "If you always do what you've always done, then you'll always get what you've always gotten." The man said, "Huh? What do you think that means?" He then jumped into the water, and as usual, the tide quickly pulled him back to the island.

The young girl watched from shore and thought about the note in the bottle. She said to the man and woman, "I've watched you day after day trying to swim to the mainland only to fail every time. The note in the bottle read, 'If you always do what you've always done, you'll always get what you've always gotten.' I think that it means that if you keep trying to swim the same way to the mainland, you'll always be pulled back to shore. To reach the mainland, I believe we need to think and do something differently than what we have been thinking and doing."

The man and woman looked at her with a condescending smile and jumped into the water to swim to the mainland only to be quickly pulled back to shore because of the strong tide.

While the man and woman continued their quest to reach the mainland, the girl gathered materials from the island. She built a raft and said to the man and woman, "I'm going to try to reach the mainland using the raft, but I'm going to set off from the other side of the island." The man and woman laughed, "You will be even farther from the mainland. You will never succeed."

Later that day, the man and woman lay on shore exhausted from being pulled back into shore after another swimming attempt to reach the mainland. They heard a call from the distance, "I'll send help!" It was the young girl. They watched as she became smaller and smaller in the distance, the distance that brought her closer and closer to the mainland.

Review and Closure

Purpose

The purpose of Review and Closure is to give participants an opportunity to analyze, synthesize, and integrate learning that occurred during the session. The Review and Closure exercises provide a means for exploring each individual's and family's growth and development, and for formulating action plans to transfer learning to other life situations.

Strategies

- ☐ Devote as much time, energy, and creativity to the design of the Review and Closure component as is devoted to the other program components.
- ☐ Allot ample time for an effective and unhurried Review and Closure.
- ☐ The Review and Closure should include activities and exercises to have participants:
  1. articulate and summarize meaningful learning,
  2. highlight and recognize accomplishments and achievements,
  3. finish any unfinished business and tie up any loose ends,
  4. celebrate and acknowledge new learning,
  5. explore how the program experiences apply to other life situations,
  6. develop postsession action plans that specify the application of new learning,
  7. discuss obstacles that may be faced when attempting to transfer new learning and describe the methods that will be used to overcome the obstacles,
  8. create support systems to monitor postprogram action plans developed by the participants and/or families, and
  9. design some techniques for providing postprogram reinforcement and boosts.

Review and Closure exercises follow.

The Family Feelings Chart

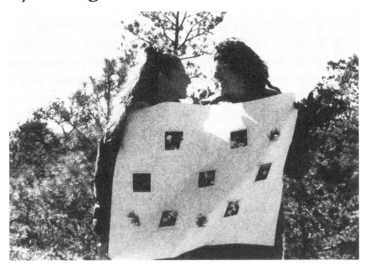

The Family Feelings Chart is a pictorial representation of emotions demonstrated by the family members. It is used to help family members identify and process how they are feeling during and after the experiential exercises.

Materials Required

- ☐ Camera & film—at least one or two rolls per family
- ☐ Poster board
- ☐ Rubber cement, glue, or tape
- ☐ Markers

Procedures

1. Take lots of pictures of the family participating in the experiential exercises. Try to to get pictures of various family configurations (i.e., individual portraits, full family, family subgroups) expressing a variety of emotions (e.g., joy, excitement, frustration, anger, hopelessness, sadness, etc.). The key is to get pictures of a variety of expressed emotions.
2. After the pictures are developed, ask the family to create their Family Feelings Chart. Have them identify the emotions being expressed in each of the pictures. Some families may not have had much experience identifying or labeling their feelings. In such a case, a commercially produced Feelings Chart (such as those sold by companies that sell therapeutic books and toys for children) can be used to assist the family. They can match the expressions from the commercial chart with those expressions demonstrated in their photographs.
3. After the family members agree what emotions are being expressed in the photograph, have them tape or glue the photograph on the poster board and label it by writing the emotion underneath the picture. The family does this for each

of the pictures, creating several rows and columns until all pictures have been identified and placed on the poster board. The creation of the Family Feelings Chart, in and of itself, can be a powerful processing tool.

4. The Family Feelings Chart can be used in future counseling sessions to assist the family in identifying their feelings. They can identify pictures from the Family Feelings Chart that match how they are feeling during and after the exercise.

Structured Questionnaires

If a family is fairly verbal and enjoys writing things down, a structured questionnaire can help the family review the session. The questionnaire should be developed and selected to match the goals of the family as well as those issues that came out during the session. Two examples, the Family Interaction Assessment and the Family Strengths Focus, follow.

Materials Required

- ☐ One questionnaire per participant
- ☐ Writing instrument

Procedures

1. Choose or create a structured questionnaire that best matches the participating family's needs and goals. See sample questions that follow.

   Questions to elicit information about family interactions.

   - ☐ Who has the responsibility for the family tasks?
   - ☐ Are you polite or angry with one another?
   - ☐ How do you react to disagreements or do you always agree?
   - ☐ Are you hopeful or do you feel helpless?
   - ☐ What are your strengths?
   - ☐ How do you show affection?
   - ☐ What positive methods of communication do you demonstrate?

   Questions to elicit information about family strengths.

   - ☐ What did your family do well during the exercises?
   - ☐ How did your family express its care and concern for one another during the exercises?
   - ☐ How did your family help one another (and the other families) during the exercises?
   - ☐ What qualities and strengths does your family have that you would not want to lose?
   - ☐ When future problems arise in your family, how will your family strengths help you solve them?

2. Distribute one copy per participant and ask them to individually complete them.
3. Lead a discussion that allows all of the family members to share their results.

Sample Questionnaires follow.

Family Interaction Assessment

Who has the responsibility for the family tasks?

Are you polite or angry with one another?

How do you react to disagreements or do you always agree?

Are you hopeful or do you feel helpless?

What are your strengths?

How do you show affection?

What positive methods of communication do you demonstrate?

Family Strengths Focus

What did your family do well during the exercises?

How did your family express its care and concern for one another during the exercises?

How did your family help one another (and the other families) during the exercises?

What qualities and strengths does your family have that you would not want to lose?

When future problems arise in your family, how will your family strengths help you solve them?

Expressive Arts Exercises for Review and Closure

Following are seven experiential, expressive arts activities that can assist with the review and closure process.

Nature Symbol

If a nature setting is near the counseling site, you can ask the family to go on a quest to locate an object in nature that represents those family strengths demonstrated during the family-building initiatives. If the symbol is transportable and does not destroy the natural environment, it should be brought back with them. If it cannot be brought back, it can verbally be described by the participants. They then should describe the symbol's significance to the counselor and other participating families.

The Family Crest

Give the family a large sheet of newsprint and a variety of different colored magic markers, colored pencils, and crayons. Their task, as a family, is to depict their family's strengths through a drawing. This may be introduced as the creation of a Family Crest—a pictorial representation of the positive things about their family, or a symbol of how they want future generations to remember them. It is important to stress that, as with the family-building initiatives, each family member should play a part in its development. After completion, give the family an opportunity to describe their Family Crest and have each family member explain how he or she contributed to its construction.

The Family Fantasy World

During the experiential exercises, take instant photographs with a Polaroid®-type camera. As a way to reinforce and bring closure to the session, give the family the pictures of their family along with scissors, newsprint, and a variety of markers or colored pencils. Tell them that their task is to construct a family fantasy world in which all their strengths and resources are available and consistently used. They are instructed to first cut out the family figures from their background in the photographs.

Ask them to use the magic markers, colored pencils, and crayons to create a background for their family picture cut-outs that depicts the optimal use of their strengths and resources. When they are finished, invite them to describe their finished project.

The Family Book

As with the Family Fantasy World exercise, take instant photographs of the family with a Polaroid-type camera. As a way to reinforce and provide closure to the session, give the family their pictures, scissors, construction paper, string or yarn, and a variety of markers or colored pencils. Give them the task to create a homemade book describing their experiences during the program. Ask them to write the story of their involvement in the program and to use their photographs and personal artwork as illustrations. A cover can be created for the book, and the pages can be held together with string or yarn that is tied through holes made with a hole punch or a pencil.

Family Warm Fuzzies

Assemble a wide variety of 3-dimensional materials including pompoms (1" to 3"), small toy eyes, pieces of felt and cardboard, and lots of white glue. Ask each family member to construct a symbol for each of their other family members. These symbols, or "warm fuzzies," should represent the other family member's strengths. Give each family member the opportunity to share their symbols and their assigned meanings with his family members.

Bead Giving

Give each member a piece of lace early in the counseling program. Keep a variety of different colored beads on hand (they can be purchased at hobby stores). When a participant does something special (anything from arriving on time to sharing something very personal to helping another group member), award them with a bead. Act as a model for bead-giving, and then encourage the other members to become the bead-givers. Don't give out beads freely, nor use them as a bribe (e.g., "If you do this, then I'll give you a bead.") This guideline helps keep the beads special.

Beads may be assigned specific meanings based on their colors. A color-coded chart that designates the meaning of the beads can be laminated and distributed to all of the participants. A example of a Bead Giving Chart follows:

- ☐ Purple = Bravery
- ☐ White = Sharing Something Pure of Heart
- ☐ Red = Doing Something Loving
- ☐ Black = Being Powerful/Strong
- ☐ Yellow = Being Warm
- ☐ Green = Personal Growth
- ☐ Blue = Giving to Others

Word for the Day

This family strength reinforcer is a good and quick session closer. Have the family members decide by consensus on one word that represents the strengths they demonstrated during the family-building initiatives. After they decide on their word, ask them to form a circle with their arms around the people next to them (in a group hug configuration). Instruct them to put their right foot in the middle of the circle with their heels on the ground and toes pointing up into the air. On the count of three, they yell out the word so the world can hear it while stomping down their right feet to ground their word.

Follow-Up Contracts

Follow-Up Contracts specify those commitments and actions the family is willing to take following the program. The Follow-Up Contract is often the most powerful tool used to facilitate the transfer of the counseling session learnings to other life situations. It specifies, in concrete and specific terms, what actions the family plans to take in the future because of their counseling experiences. Because it is written, it becomes a powerful visual reminder to the family members of their commitments to one another and their family unit.

Materials Required

- ☐ One contract per participant or per family (depending on the needs and desires of the family and counselor)
- ☐ Pencils or pens

Sample

A sample contract follows. It asks the family to:

- ☐ review their experience and choose a significant learning,
- ☐ specify behaviors that they will stop, continue, and start due to their experience,
- ☐ identify a method for assessing progress, and
- ☐ describe how they will celebrate progress made on their contract.

Procedures

1. Discuss with the family if they would like to complete the Follow-Up Contract individually or as a family unit.
2. After completing the contract, ask the family participants how they plan to follow-up on the contract. If working in a multifamily group format, the following strategies can be used:

   - ☐ The families can exchange contracts at the end of the session. These can be mailed back to the contract creators several weeks later with a note of encouragement.
   - ☐ Families can contact one another by telephone at predetermined intervals to discuss progress on the contract.
   - ☐ A progress meeting can be scheduled several weeks following the completion of the program. During that meeting, families can report on progress made on their contract.

Contract With Ourselves

Our most significant learning, for our family, during the experience was:

We plan to incorporate this information into our lives by

☐ starting to

☐ stopping

☐ continuing to

We plan to assess our progress by

We plan to celebrate our progress by

Signature(s): _____ Date: _____

BIBLIOGRAPHY

Berg, I. K. (1994). *Family based services: A solution-focused approach.* New York: W. W. Norton.

Bettelheim, B. (March, 1987). The importance of play. *The Atlantic, 259.*

Brendtro, L., Brokenleg, M., & Van Bockern, S. (1990). *Reclaiming youth at risk: Our hope for the future.* Bloomington, IL: National Educational Service.

Buckley, M. R., Thorngren, J. M., & Kleist, D. M. (1997). Family resiliency: A neglected family construct. *The Family Journal: Counseling and Therapy for Couples and Families, 5,* 241–246.

Chase, N. K. (1981). *Outward Bound in the treatment of alcoholism.* Denver, CO: Colorado Outward Bound School. (ERIC Document Reproduction Service No. ED 241 204).

Chethik, M. (1989). *Techniques of child therapy: Psychodynamic strategies.* New York: The Guilford Press.

Clapp, C. L., & Rudolph, S. M. (1993). Building family teams: An adventure-based approach to enrichment and intervention. In M. A. Gass (Ed.), *Adventure Therapy: Therapeutic Applications of Adventure Programming* (pp. 111-121). Dubuque, IA: Kendall-Hunt.

Croake, J. W. (1983). Adlerian parent education. *The Counseling Psychologist, 11*(3), 65–70.

Davis, D. (1987). *Alcoholism treatment.* New York: Gardner.

Dr. Suess. (1996). *My many colored days.* New York: Alfred A. Knopf.

Eaker, B. (1994). Unlocking the family secret in family play therapy. In C. Schaefer & L. Carey (Ed.), *Family play therapy* (pp. 107–126). Northvale, NJ: Jason Aronson.

Eastwood, M., Sweeney, D., & Piercy, F. (1987). The "no-problem problem": A family therapy approach for certain first time adolescent substance abusers. *Family Relations, 36,* 125–128.

Fatis, M., & Konewko, P. J. (1983, March-April). Written contracts as adjuncts in family therapy. *Social Work,* 161–163.

Fishman, H. C., Stanton, M. D., Roseman, B. L. (1982). Treating families of adolescent drug abusers. In M. D. Stanton and T. C. Todd (Eds.), *Strategies and techniques of treatment.* New York: Guildford.

Fluegelman, A. (1981). *More new games.* New York: Doubleday & Co.

Fluegelman, A. (1976). *The new games book.* New York: Doubleday & Co.

Freeman, J., Epston, D., & Lobotvits, D. (1997). *Playful approaches to serious problems.* New York: W. W. Norton.

Garcia-Preto, N. (1989). Transformation of the family system in adolescence. In B. Carter, & M. McGoldrick (Eds.), *The changing family life cycle: A framework for family therapy* (2nd ed.). Boston: Allyn & Bacon.

Gass, M. A. (1993). Foundations of adventure therapy. In M. A. Gass (Ed.), *Adventure therapy: Therapeutic applications of adventure programming* (pp. 3–10). Dubuque, IA: Kendall-Hunt.

Gass, M. A., & Scippa, M. (1990). Enhancing therapeutic adventure experiences through the use of prescriptive metaphors. In R. F. Flor (Ed.), *1990 Conference of the Association for Experiential Education* (pp. 90–93). Boulder, CO: Association for Experiential Education.

Gerstein, J. S. (1998). *A place of connection: Expressive counseling activities for individuals and families.* Oklahoma City: Wood 'N' Barnes.

Gerstein, J. (1997). *Living metaphors: Stories and experiential exercises for individual, group, and family growth.* Dubuque, IL: Kendall-Hunt.

Gerstein, J. S. (1996). Case study invited response. In J. L. Luckner & R. S. Nadler, *Processing the experience: Strategies to enhance and generalize learning* (pp. 289–294). Dubuque, IA: Kendall-Hunt.

Gil, E. (1994). *Play in family therapy*. New York: The Guildford Press.

Gillis, H. L., & Gass, M. (1993). Bringing adventure into marriage and family therapy: An innovative experiential approach. *Journal of Marital and Family Therapy, 19,* 273–286.

Gillis, H. L., & Gass, M. (1991). *An overview of adventure experiences used in marriage and family therapy.* Unpublished Manuscript.

Gregson, B. (1984). *The outrageous outdoor games book.* Belmont, CA: Pitman Learning, Inc.

Haley, J. (1976). *Problem-solving therapy.* New York: Harper Books.

Heath, A. W. & Ayers, T. C. (1988). *MRI brief therapy with adolescent substance abusers.* Unpublished Manuscript.

Huber, C. H. (1997). Outward bound together (indoors): Adventure family counseling. *The Family Journal: Counseling and Therapy for Couples and Families, 5,* 49–52.

Irwin, E. C., & Malloy, E. S. (1994). Family puppet interview. In C. Schaefer & L. Carey (Ed.), *Family play therapy* (pp. 21–34). Northvale, NJ: Jason Aronson.

Jurich, A. P., Polson, C. J., Jurich, J. A., & Bates, R. A. (1985). Family factors in the lives of drug users and abusers. *Adolescence, 20,* 143–155.

Kimball, R. O. (1983). The wilderness as therapy. *Journal of Experiential Education, 5,* 6–9.

Luckner, J. L., & Nadler, R. S. (1997). *Processing the experience: Strategies to enhance and generalize learning.* Dubuque, IA: Kendall-Hunt.

Madanas, C. (1981). *Strategic family therapy.* San Francisco: Jossey-Bass.

Markowitz, L. (July/August, 1997) A kid's eye view of therapy. *The Family Therapy Networker,* pp. 32–33.

McHardy, J., & Root, K. (1992). Adventure based family counselling. In G. M. Hanna (Ed.), *Proceedings of the 20th Annual AEE Conference* (pp. 130–131). Boulder, CO: Association for Experiential Education.

Miller, W. (1994). Family play therapy: History, theory, and convergence. In C. Schaefer & L. Carey (Eds.), *Family play therapy* (pp. 3–20). Northvale, NJ: Jason Aronson.

O'Hanlon, W. (in press). *A field guide to possibility land.*

Quereau, T. (1993, Fall). Play in counseling. *American Counselor,* pp. 9–13.

Riley, S. (1994). *Integrative approaches to family art therapy.* Chicago, IL: Magnolia Street Publishers.

Rohnke, K. (1984). *Silver bullets: A guide to initiative problems, adventure games, stunts, and trust activities.* Hamilton, MA: Project Adventure.

Rosenthal, H. G. (1998). *Favorite counseling and therapy techniques.* Philadelphia, PA: Accelerated Development.

Rudolph, S. (1997). Families on the ropes: Programming with families. In J. L. Luckner & R. S. Nadler, *Processing the Experience* (pp. 274–282). Dubuque, IA: Kendall-Hunt Publishers.

Satir, V. (1964). *Conjoint family therapy.* Palo Alto: Science and Behavior Books.

Simon, R. (November, December, 1994). Psychotherapy's third wave? The promise of narrative. *Family Therapy Networker,* p. 2.

Stanton, M. D. (1981). Family treatment approaches to drug problems: A review. *Family Process, 18,* 251–280.

Stanton, M. D. & Todd, T. C. (1982). *Strategies and Techniques of Treatment.* New York: Guildford.

Stitch, T. F. (1983). Experiential therapy for psychiatric patients. *Journal of Experiential Education, 5,* 23–30.

Stitch, T. F., & Senior, N. (1984). Adventure therapy: An innovative treatment for psychiatric patients. In B. Pepper & H. Ryglewicz (Eds.), *New Directions for Mental Health Services* (No. 21). San Francisco, CA: Jossey-Bass.

Stone, S., McKay, M. M., & Stoops, C. (1996). Evaluating multiple family groups to address the behavioral difficulties of urban children. *Small Group Research, 27,* 398–415.

Thorngren, J. M., Christensen, T. M., & Kleist, D. M. (1998). Multi-family group treatment: The under explored therapy. *The Family Journal: Counseling and Therapy for Couples and Families, 6,* 125–131.

Vass, M., Jacobs, E., & Slavek, N. (1984). Live-in family counseling: An integrated approach. *The Personnel and Guidance Journal,* 429–431.

Weider, R. (1979). Viewing Outward Bound as an experience based counseling model. In B. Harris & D. K. Wilson (Eds.), *Adventure programs for human services.* Denver, CO: Colorado Outward Bound School.

Weinstein, M., & Goodman, J. (1980). *Playfair.* San Luis Obispo, CA: Impact Publishers.

Wick, D. T., Wick, J. K., & Peterson, N. (1997). Improving self-esteem with Adlerian adventure therapy. *Professional School Counseling, 1,* 53–56.

Winnicott, D.W. (1965). *The maturational process and the facilitating environment.* New York: International Universities Press.

Wood, A. (1982). *Quick as a cricket.* Child's Play International.

Zilbach, J. J. (1994). *Young children in family therapy.* Northvale, NJ: Jason Aronson, Inc.

Zimmerman, J. J. (1992). *Make Beliefs.* New York: Bantam Books.

AUTHOR INDEX

A
Ayers, T. C., 105, 106

B
Berg, I. K., 23, 105
Bettelheim, B., 169
Brendtro, L., 40
Brokenleg, M., 40
Buckley, M. R., 4

C
Chase, 81, 3
Christensen, T. M., 5
Clapp, C. L., 2, 14

D
Davis, D., 12, 23, 105
Dr. Seuss, 169

E
Eaker, B., 7
Eastwood, M., 11, 25, 31
Epson, D., 4, 7, 25, 26

F
Fatis, M., 71
Fishman, H. C., 12
Freeman, J., 4, 7, 25, 26
Fluegelman, A., 97

G
Garcia-Preto, N., 38
Gass, M. A., 2, 3, 4, 27, 29, 31, 105
Gerstein, J., 4, 28, 29
Gillis, H. L., 3, 27, 29, 31, 105
Goodman, J., 89
Green, R. J., 7
Griego, G., 127

H
Hahn, K., 1
Haley, J., 23, 105
Heath, A. W., 105, 106
Huber, C. H., 2

I
Irwin, E. C., 9
Itin, C., 117

J
Jacobs, E., 5

K
Kleist, D. M., 4, 5
Konewko, P. J., 71

L
Lobovits, D., 4, 7, 25, 26
Luckner, J. L., 2, 106

M
Madanas, C., 34
Malloy, E. S., 9
Markowitz, L., 34
McHardy, J., 13
McKay, M. M., 5
Miller, W., 8, 9

N–O
Nadler, R. S., 2, 106
Norton, B., 94
O'Hanlon, W., 23, 105, 106

P–Q
Peterson, N., 2, 8
Piercy, F., 11, 25, 31
Quereau, T., 7

R
Riley, S., 6
Rohnke, K., 1
Root, K., 13
Roseman, B. L., 12
Rosenthal, H. G., 8
Rudolph, S., 2, 5, 11, 12, 14, 27

S
Satir, V., 34
Scippa, M., 2
Simon, R., 6
Slavek, N., 5
Stanton, M. D., 5, 11, 12, 106
Stitch, T. F., 1, 105
Stone, S., 5
Stoops, C., 5
Sweeney, D., 11, 25, 31

T
Thorngren, J. M., 4, 5, 98
Todd, T. C., 11, 12, 106

V
Van Bockern, S., 40
Vass, M., 5

W
Webb, B., 117
Weinstein, M., 89
Wick, D. T., 2, 8
Wick, J. K., 2, 8
Winnicott, D. W., 35
Wood, A., 170

Z
Zimmerman, J. J., 71

SUBJECT INDEX

A

Abuse
  and family knots game, 119
  and family pick-up sticks game, 114
Acceptable/unacceptable behaviors form, 73
Acting, as metaphor, 9
Action-centered family counseling, 4
Adjunct programs, 28
Adventure education, 1
Alcohol-related issues, 10
American Psychological Association, code of ethics
    of, 17
Arts and crafts
  in chain reaction game, 127–128
  in T-shirt panorama, 147
Arts exercises, for review and closure, 163–164
Asking for help, in family jewels game, 122–123
Attention span, of young children, 35
Audio-visual recordings, 19

B

Background information, 19
Barrier break down, family-building initiatives for, 104
Beach ball toss, 93
  follow-up questions for, 94
Behavior testing, 9–10
Behavioral contracts, 75
  steps in, 71
Behaviors, negative, identification of, 127–128
Behaviors form, 73
Biblio check-in, 57

C

Chain reaction, 127–128
Challenged children, 37
Change, of family patterns, 9–10
Children. See also Experiential family counseling,
    young children in
  behavioral contracts for, 71–77
  developmental needs in, 7–8

Code of ethics, 17
Communication
  to adolescents, 39–40
  in counseling session, 10–11
  in family knots exercise, 117–118
Competition, on children, 36
Confidentiality, 19
Contracts, 67–77
  behavioral, 75
  behavioral, steps in, 71
  behaviors form in, 73
  definition of, 67
  family, 69
  family, sample of, 77
  follow-up, in experimental program setup, 31
  followup, in review and closure, 165
  with ourselves, in review and closure, 167
Cooperation
  in dumping field game, 143
  in family jewels game, 122–123
  illustration of, 111
Counseling, experiential family. See Experiential
    family counseling
Counseling session, 43–167
  contracts for, 67–77 (See also Contracts)
  experiential check-in activities for, 51–61 (See also
    Experiential check-in activities)
  family-building initiatives in, 101–151 (See also
    Family-building initiatives)
  goals of, 43
  interest and motivation for, 8
  name games in, 79–85 (See also Name games)
  participant bill of rights in, 65
  participant responsibilities in, 66
  participant rights and responsibilities in, 63
  PEEP in, 44–49 (See also PEEP)
  review and closure in, 153–167 (See also Review
    and closure, of counseling session)
  safety check for, physical and emotional, 43–44
  warm-ups in, 79, 87–100 (See also Warm-ups)

Crossing over hard ships, 139–141
   processing of, 142
Crossing the Problem Pit, 9–10, 135–138
Cultural issues, of young children, 36–37

D
Desert island, 149–151
Developmental issues
   of adolescents, 38
   of children, 35–36
Duck, duck, goose name game, 83
Dumping field, 143–146

E
Education, adventure, 1
Emotional risk, informed consent for, 20
Emotional safety check, 43–45, 49
Environmental check, 45, 49
Experiential activities, function of, 8–10
Experiential check-in activities, 51–61
   biblio check-in as, 57
   movement chain as, 53
   musical feelings as, 55
   pick a feeling as, 61
   puppet check-in as, 59
Experiential family counseling
   counseling session in (*See* Counseling session)
   follow-up strategies for, 31
   preparation for, 13–25 (*See also* Experiential
      family counseling, experimental program setup
      in)
   program for, 27–29
Experiential family counseling, adolescents in, 38–
      42
   art and music in, 41
   developmental issues of, 38
   gender and sexual orientation in, 40–41
   guiding metaphor in, 41–42
   humor in, 41
   leadership opportunities for, 39
   positive communication in, 39–40
   power struggles in, 40
   resistance in, 40
Experiential family counseling, experimental
      program setup in, 13–31
   adjunct programs in, 28
   assessment in, 28–29
   community-based programs in, 27
   family interests and strengths inventory in, 25–26
   family performance agreement in, 14–15
   family performance commitment in, 16
   follow-up contracts in, 31
   goal checklist in, 25
   goal setting and problem description in, 23
   goal setting recommendations in, 23
   informed consent in, 17–21
   meeting times in, convenience of, 27–28
   participant registration in, 17–21
   participant selection in, 13–14

program orientation in, 13–14
progress meetings in, 28
services menu in, 28
Experiential family counseling, foundations of, 1–12
   acting as metaphor in, 9
   action-centered, 4
   behavior testing in, 9–10
   children's developmental needs in, 7–8 (*See also*
      Experiential family counseling, young children
      in)
   communication in, 10–11
   counseling session in, interest and motivation for,
      8
   definition of, 1–3
   family pattern change in, 9–10
   family roles in, 12
   information generation in, 9
   multi-family groups in, 5–6
   narrative therapy approach in, 6
   naturalistic interaction, 4–5
   play focus in, 6–7, 12
   resistance reduction in, 8
   solution-focused orientation in, 11–12
   strength identification in, 11
   strength-promoting, 4
Experiential family counseling, young children in,
      34–37
   attention span in, 35
   challenged children in, 37
   cultural issues in, 36–37
   multi-family groups in, 36
   orientation for, 34–35
   skills in, physical and verbal, 35–36
Experiential program set-up, 13–31. See also
      Experiential family counseling, experiential
      program setup of
Expressive arts exercises, for review and closure,
      163–164

F
Family, healthy *vs.* unhealthy communication in,
      117–118
Family-building initiatives, 101–151
   chain reaction as, 127–128
   crossing over hard ships as, 139–142
   crossing the problem pit as, 135–138
   desert island as, 149–151
   dumping field as, 143–146
   family jewels as, 121–123
   family juggle as, 107–108
   family knots as, 117–119
   family obstacle field as, 133–134
   family parts as, 115–116
   family pick-up sticks as, 113–114
   family strengths protector as, 129–131
   family tower of power as, 125
   nurturing spoons as, 109–110
   nurturing spoons as, story of, 111
   purpose of, 101

selection guidelines for, 103
strategies for using, 104–106
T-shirt panorama as, 147
Family commitment, in family performance
agreement, 16
Family contracts, 69. *See also* Contracts
sample of, 77
Family counseling, experiential. *See* Experiential
family counseling
Family feelings chart, 155–156
Family "have you evers," 87
questions for, 88
Family interaction assessment, 159
Family jewels, 121–123
Family juggle, 107–108
Family jump rope, 95
Family knots, 117–119
Family obstacle field, 133–134
Family parts, 115–116
Family pattern change, 9–10
Family performance agreement, 14–15
Family performance commitment, 16
Family pick-up sticks, 113–114
Family scavenger hunt, 89
Family strengths
focus on, in review and closure, 161
goals of experiential family counseling, 25
identification of, 105
identification of, family tower of power for, 125
inventory of family interests and strengths, 25
Family strengths protector, 129–131
Family tower of power, 125
Family we-play, 97
Follow-up contracts
in experimental program setup, 31
in review and closure, 165
Fun, 6–7, 12
in family-building initiatives, 104–105
goals of experiential family counseling, 25

G
Gender and sexual orientation, of adolescents, 40–41
Goal checklist, 25
Goals
checklist for, 25
of counseling session, 43
of experiential family counseling, 10–12
setting of, 23
therapeutic, 10–12
Group games. *See* Family-building initiatives
Group power, 109

H
Hard ships, crossing over, 139–142
"Have you evers" warm-up exercise, 87
questions for, 88
Hierarchy, in family systems, 133–134
goals of experiential family counseling, 25
Human scavenger hunt, 90

Humor, 7

I
Incest, and family pick-up sticks game, 114
Information generation, 9
Informed consent, sample forms for, 17–21
Initiatives, family-building, 101–151. *See also* Family-
building initiatives
Interactions, naturalistic, 4–5
Inventory, of family interests and strengths, 25–26

J
Juggling, as family-building initiative, 107–108
Jump rope, 95

L
Leadership opportunities, for adolescents, 39
Learning, cyclical model of, 2

M
Make beliefs, 99–100
Medical care authorization, 20
Metaphors
acting as, 9
for adolescent counseling, 41–42
family-building initiatives as, 105
of family experience, family knots in, 117
of life experience, family jewels in, 121
Movement chain, 53
Multi-family groups
counseling of, 5–6
young children in, 36
Multi-session format, 27
Musical feelings, 55

N
Name games, 79–85
duck, duck, goose, 83
other side of the blanket, 85
purpose and strategy of, 79
toss a name, 81
Narrative therapy approach, 6
Naturalistic interactions, 4–5
Nurturing spoons, 109–110
story of, 111

O
Obstacle field, 133–134
Orientation, for young children, 34–35
Other side of the blanket, 85

P
Parent, and adolescent power struggles, 40
Parental permission, in participant registration, 20
Participant
bill of rights for, 65
registration of, 17–21
Participant responsibilities, 66
in family performance agreement, 15

Participant rights and responsibilities, 63
Participant selection, in experimental program
    setup, 13–14
Pattern change, of family, 9–10
Patterns, breaking of, 108
PEEP (physical, emotional, environmental, and
        personal check), 44–49
    as intervention, 47
    methodology of, 46–47
    normalizing in, 47
    safety check in, 44–46
    safety checklist in, 49
    stop mechanism in, 44–46
Penny for your thoughts, 91
    questions for, 92
Performance agreement, 14–15
Performance commitment, 16
Personal check, 45–46, 49
Physical risk, informed consent for, 20
Physical safety check, 43–45, 49
Physical skills, of children, 35–36
Pick a feeling, 61
Pick-up sticks, family, 113–114
Play, in experiential family counseling, 6–7, 12
Positive communication, to adolescents, 39–40
Power struggles, with adolescents, 40
Privacy, 19
Problem behaviors, identification of, chain reaction
        game for, 127–128
Problem Pit, crossing of, 9–10, 135–138
Problematic patterns
    identification and disruption of, 106
    identification of, crossing the Problem Pit in,
        135–138
Processing session, after family-building initiatives, 106
Program activities, in family performance agree-
        ment, 15
Program orientation, in experimental program
        setup, 13–14
Program services, in family performance agreement,
        15
Program setup, 13–31. *See also* Experiential family
        counseling, experiential program setup
Progress meetings, 28
Puppet check-in, 59

Q
Questionnaires, for review and closure, 157

R
Registration, sample forms for, 17–21
Resistance
    of adolescents, 40
    reduction of, 8
Review and closure, of counseling session, 153–167
    contracts in, follow-up, 165
    contracts in, with ourselves, 167
    expressive arts exercises in, 163–164

family feelings chart in, 155–156
family interaction assessment in, 159
family strengths focus in, 161
purpose of, 153
questionnaires in, structured, 157
strategies for, 153
Rights, of participants. *See* participant rights and
    responsibilities
Risk, informed consent for, 19–20

S
Safety, in family-building initiatives, 104
Safety check, 43–46
    checklist for, 49
Scavenger hunt
    family, 89
    human, 90
Sexual orientation, of adolescents, 40–41
Skills level, of young children, 35–36
Solution, *vs.* problem emphasis, 105
Stop mechanism, of PEEP, 46
Strength, identification of
    in counseling, 11
    family-building initiatives in, 105
    family tower of power for, 125
Strengths
    focus on, in review and closure, 161
    promotion of, 4
Stress, on family system, 129–130

T
T-shirt panorama, 147
Teamwork
    in crossing over hardships, 139–141
    in family parts, 115–116
    in family pick-up sticks, 113–114
Therapeutic goals and principles, 10–12
Time-outs, 104
Toss a name, 81
Tower of power, 125

V
Verbal skills, of children, 35–36

W
Warm-ups, 79, 87–100
    beach ball toss, 93
    beach ball toss, follow-up questions for, 94
    family "have you evers," 87
    family "have you evers," questions for, 88
    family jump rope, 95
    family scavenger hunt, 89
    family we-play, 97
    human scavenger hunt, 90
    make beliefs, 99–100
    penny for your thoughts, 91
    penny for your thoughts, questions for, 92
We-play, 97

T - #0704 - 101024 - C0 - 276/216/10 - PB - 9781560328643 - Gloss Lamination